Balance Exercises
for Better Bones

Grace Vinson

COPYRIGHT

In no way is it legal to reproduce, duplicate, or transmit any part of this document electronically or in printed format. The recording of this publication is strictly prohibited. Any storage of this document is not allowed unless with written permission from the publisher. All rights reserved.

The information provided herein is stated to be truthful and consistent. In terms of inattention or otherwise, any liability, by any use or abuse of any policies, processes, or directions contained within is the solitary and utter responsibility of the recipient reader. Under no circumstances will any reparation, damages, or monetary loss due to the information herein, either directly or indirectly.

Disclaimer Notice: Please note the information contained within this document is for educational and entertainment purposes only. Every attempt has been made to provide accurate, up-to-date, reliable, complete information. However, no warranties of any kind are expressed or implied. The reader acknowledges that the author does not render legal, financial, medical, or professional advice. The content of this book has been derived from various sources. Please consult a licensed professional before attempting any techniques outlined in this book.

NOTE: This manual is in no way intended as a substitute for specific medical care.

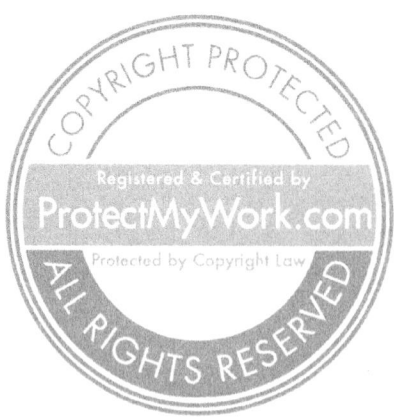

Copyright Protected with www.ProtectMyWork.com

Table of Contents

Introduction 5

Signs of Declining Balance 6

Delving into Balance Dynamics and Causes 8

Navigating Balance Issues: What to Do 10

Exploring Natural Solutions for Balance Enhancement 11

EYE EXERCISES 12

Ocular training 13

Peripheral ocular focus 14

Ocular Dissociation 15

Arm-Eye coordination 16

Advanced arm-Eye coordination 17

BALANCE EXERCISES 19

Sit to Stand 20

Tip-toe Balance 22

Advanced Tip-toe Balance 24

Basic Toe Balance 26

Advanced Toe Balance 28

Toe-Heel Balance 30

Tip-toe Walk 32

Heel Walk 34

Baby Steps 36

March Steps 38

Side Leg Raise 40

Leg Lift 42

Advanced Leg Lift 44

Single-Leg Balance 46

Advanced Single-Leg Balance 48

Back Leg Extensions 50

Knee Flex and Lift 52

Toe-to-Knee Chair Assisted 54

Ankle Point and Flex 56

Advanced Leg Hold Balance 58

Dynamic Lunge 60

28-DAY PLAN 62

Visual Warm-Up 63

Improving Awareness Exercise 64

WEEK 1 66

WEEK 2 69

WEEK 3 72

WEEK 4 75

Conclusion 79

Introduction

If you're reading these words, it's likely that you're encountering a phase in life where maintaining balance and stability feels a bit more challenging. You may have observed that simple tasks such as walking or rising from a chair demand increased effort and attention.
Rest assured, you're not alone in navigating through these changes.

As we age, our bodies undergo transformations that can affect our ability to remain steady on our feet. Muscles may lose strength, eyesight may diminish, and a variety of other factors can contribute to a sense of unsteadiness. It's as if the ground beneath us isn't as dependable as it once was, leaving us more vulnerable to stumbling.

It's no surprise that the risk of falls and injuries tends to increase as we age.
Bones become more fragile, and what might have been a minor incident in the past could now lead to significant harm, such as hip or spine fractures.

However, we don't need to simply accept these challenges. There are strategies and steps we can take to reduce the risk of falls and regain confidence in our movements.

In this book, my goal is to offer you a practical and straightforward guide to balance exercises.

These exercises are specifically tailored to enhance balance, stability, and muscle strength, particularly for seniors.

Signs of Declining Balance

Take a moment to consider your physical well-being as you review the following list. Have you experienced any of these symptoms?

- Feeling unsteady or dizzy, especially when transitioning from sitting to standing.
- Struggling to coordinate movements, particularly if you're feeling fatigued.
- Sensing instability while walking.
- Experiencing unexpected falls or loss of balance over minor obstacles like steps.
- Muscle and joint weakness or pain hindering your ability to move and walk comfortably.
- Declining vision and hearing, making it difficult to navigate your surroundings.
- Feeling disoriented, especially in unfamiliar places.
- Having trouble with positional changes, such as getting in and out of bed.
- Living with a persistent fear of falling, which may lead to constant anxiety and limited mobility.
- Dealing with ongoing tiredness and fatigue, even after several hours of waking up, often requiring frequent rest breaks.

If any of these situations resonate with you, it's likely that your balance may be compromised. However, there's no need to feel overwhelmed or anxious.

Many individuals facing similar challenges have successfully improved their situations in a relatively short period. In the upcoming chapters, we'll explore some strategies and techniques that could help you regain stability and confidence in your movements.

The best part?

You don't have to be a fitness enthusiast or invest in costly equipment to reap the benefits of these exercises. With consistent effort and a bit of practice, you'll likely notice notable improvements in.

I understand that the prospect of exercising may seem daunting, especially if you've had previous negative experiences or feel uncertain about your abilities. However, I want to reassure you that the exercise routines outlined in this book are accessible to everyone, with options to adjust difficulty levels and progress gradually.

And remember, you don't need any fancy equipment to get started.

I invite you to embark on this journey toward improved balance and enhanced confidence in your movements. With determination and dedication, we can overcome the challenges associated with aging and lead active, fulfilling lives.

Aging is a natural aspect of life that shouldn't cause undue worry.
Let's embrace the beauty of each stage of life and courageously confront the obstacles that come our way. It's time to step forward with renewed confidence and face the future head-on.

Delving into Balance Dynamics and Causes

Maintaining equilibrium relies on two primary mechanisms within our body:

- **Visual Perception:** Our eyes play a crucial role in preserving balance by providing information about our body's position relative to the surrounding environment. Closing your eyes while moving or standing demonstrates the challenge of maintaining balance without visual cues.
- **Sensory Feedback:** Sensations from our feet and other body parts in contact with the ground contribute to our awareness and stability. For seniors, utilizing a cane provides additional support by increasing points of contact with the ground, compensating for reduced strength and enhancing stability.

Understanding what contributes to a loss of balance is crucial. It's important to distinguish between factors stemming from natural physical decline and those resulting from once-functional actions that have become problematic over time. Making simple daily adjustments can yield significant overall benefits.

Take a moment to review the following list and identify any habits you may recognize in yourself that can be modified.

- **Are you leading a sedentary lifestyle?** Lack of physical activity can accelerate the deterioration of your physical condition and exacerbate issues with balance and coordination. It's essential to incorporate some form of physical activity into your routine.
- **Do you prioritize regular health assessments?** Regular health checkups are essential for maintaining balance. Monitoring vision, hearing, and blood pressure is crucial. Impairments in these areas can significantly affect balance. Schedule routine checkups to identify and address any issues early. This proactive approach helps ensure optimal sensory and cardiovascular health, reducing the risk of balance loss.
- **Do you maintain a balanced diet and hydration?** Ensuring a balanced diet and adequate hydration are essential for preserving physical well-being and promoting balance. Consuming excessive amounts of fat and sugar can negatively impact your health and disrupt your balance. Be mindful of your dietary choices to support overall health.

Additionally, proper hydration is vital for maintaining optimal physical function. Dehydration can lead to fatigue, increasing the risk of falls. Make a commitment to drink more water throughout the day to support hydration levels and enhance overall well-being.

- **Are you experiencing feelings of sadness or stress?** Mental well-being plays a crucial role in maintaining self-confidence and resilience in the face of age-related challenges. Engage in enjoyable activities to promote a healthy mindset and emotional balance.
- **Is your living environment optimized to prevent falls?** Ensuring that your home is a safe space is essential for reducing the risk of falls and enhancing overall stability. Consider evaluating your surroundings for potential hazards such as uneven surfaces and slippery floors. Implementing simple modifications like installing grab bars in bathrooms and near staircases, securing rugs to prevent tripping, and improving lighting in dimly lit areas can greatly enhance safety. Additionally, maintaining clutter-free pathways and arranging furniture to provide clear pathways can further minimize the risk of accidents.

Taking proactive measures to create a secure living environment is key to promoting safety and confidence in daily activities.

In life, experiencing both physical and mental changes is natural. Embrace these changes with tranquility and a positive attitude. Every stage of life presents its own challenges and joys, and by facing them with serenity and resilience, we can navigate through life's journey with confidence and grace.

Navigating Balance Issues: What to Do

Encountering moments of imbalance requires swift action to minimize potential risks and ensure safety. Here's a practical guide to help you handle these situations calmly and effectively:

- If you suddenly feel unsteady while standing, it's important to halt any further movement immediately. This action helps prevent a potential fall by giving you the chance to assess the situation and avoid making it worse.
- When feeling unsteady, seek stable support from nearby objects like a sturdy chair or solid furniture to regain your balance. Holding onto something secure provides immediate stability and reassurance, reducing the risk of falling.
- To manage balance issues effectively, remember to stay calm and focus on your breathing. Taking slow, deep breaths and maintaining a calm demeanor can help center yourself and reduce tension, especially when anxiety or stress exacerbates balance challenges.
- After regaining stability, take time to reflect on potential triggers for the imbalance. Consider factors such as specific activities or movements, the time of day, and any accompanying symptoms like sweating or nausea. Identifying these triggers can offer insights into your balance challenges and enable you to take preventive measures.
- Think about possible contributors to your balance challenges in your daily life. Factors such as hunger, thirst, medication side effects, recent dietary or exercise changes, and recent illnesses or injuries could all play a role. Addressing these contributors is essential for improving balance and preventing future incidents.

Exploring Natural Solutions for Balance Enhancement

Discover natural approaches to address balance loss and promote well-being:

- **Prioritize Essential Vitamins**: Ensure sufficient intake of vitamins B and D, crucial for emotional well-being and mood regulation. A balanced diet, such as the DASH DIET, rich in nutrients and low in sodium, can support overall health and aid in maintaining stability.
- **Embrace Relaxation Techniques**: Incorporate stress-reduction strategies into your routine to promote relaxation and mental clarity. Consider engaging in SOMATIC EXERCISES or meditation practices to alleviate tension and enhance resilience.

In this book, our focus will be on providing a series of exercises suitable for both standing (with optional support) and sitting positions. These exercises will progress gradually, tailored to accommodate beginners as well as those seeking to advance their balance skills to an elite level for their age. By following the guidance provided in the subsequent chapters, individuals of all abilities can regain confidence and vitality in their movements, whether walking, bending, or engaging in daily activities.

Access Exclusive Bonuses: Scan the QR code on page 18 to unlock special bonuses.

EYE EXERCISES

As we have already discussed, our vision plays a pivotal role in maintaining balance and stability, particularly as we age. Clear and coordinated vision enables us to accurately perceive our surroundings, judge distances, and react swiftly to changes in our environment, all of which are essential for maintaining equilibrium. However, age-related changes in vision can pose challenges to our balance.

To address these challenges and improve overall balance, incorporating targeted eye exercises into our daily routine is crucial. These exercises focus on enhancing visual coordination and integrating motor skills, ultimately supporting better balance and stability.

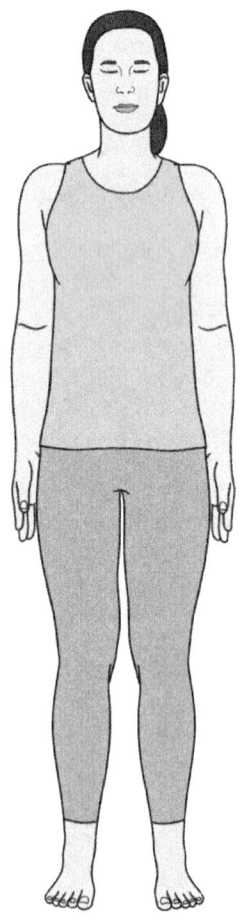

First off, stand in a stable position, ensuring your back is straight and your shoulders are relaxed. Once you feel grounded and calm, close your eyes and take deep breaths. Briefly open your eyes, then close them again.

Ocular training

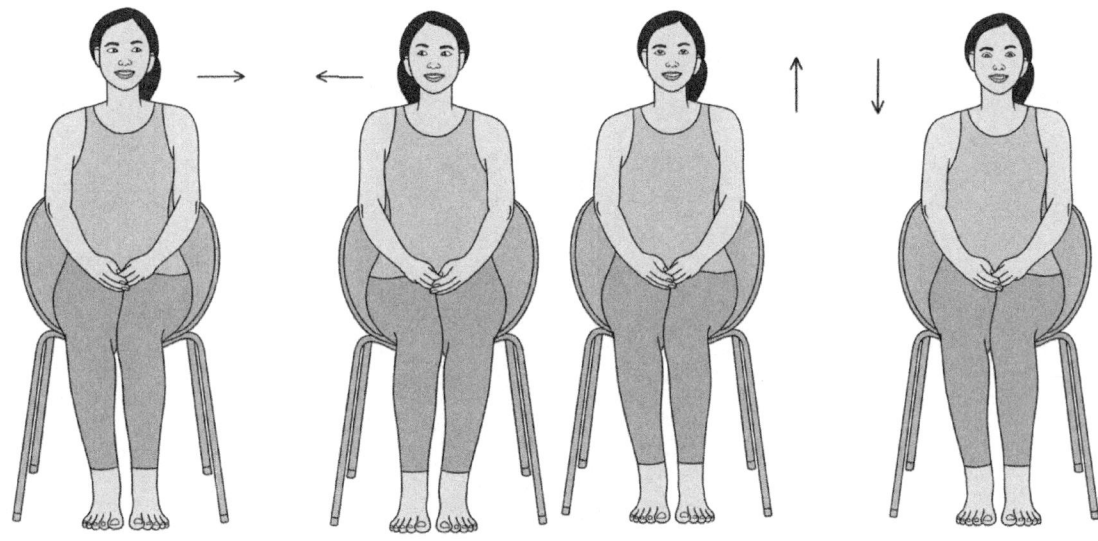

- Sit comfortably in a chair, with hands resting on your legs and maintaining a straight back.
- Keep your eyes open and your head still.
- Execute slow, repeated movements by looking up and then down, followed by slow, alternating glances to the right and left.
- Take a short break before proceeding to the next activity.

Peripheral ocular focus

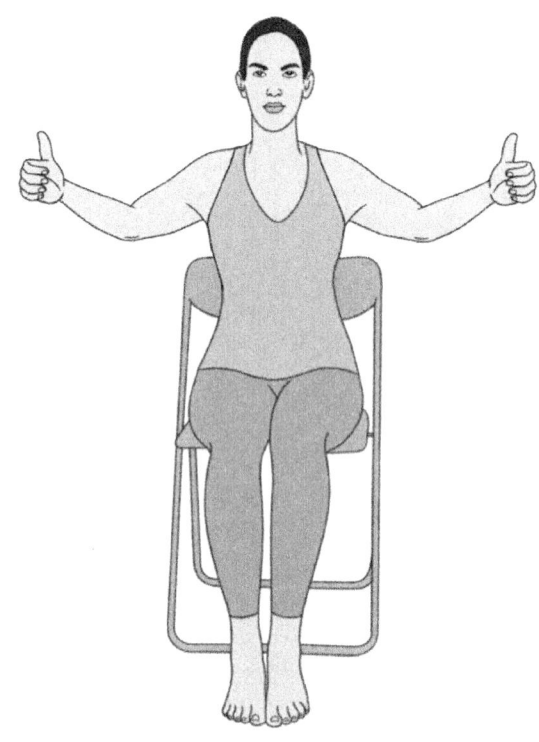

- Sit comfortably in a chair and extend your arms straight out in front of you, keeping them stretched.
- Move your arms outward until your thumbs are no longer visible in your field of vision.
- Without moving your head, focus on your right thumb, bringing it into sharp clarity, then shift your gaze to your left thumb using only your eyes.
- Increase the speed of the exercise, ensuring you maintain focus on one thumb before transitioning to the other.

This exercise aids in enhancing your peripheral vision, a crucial element for maintaining balance.

Ocular Dissociation

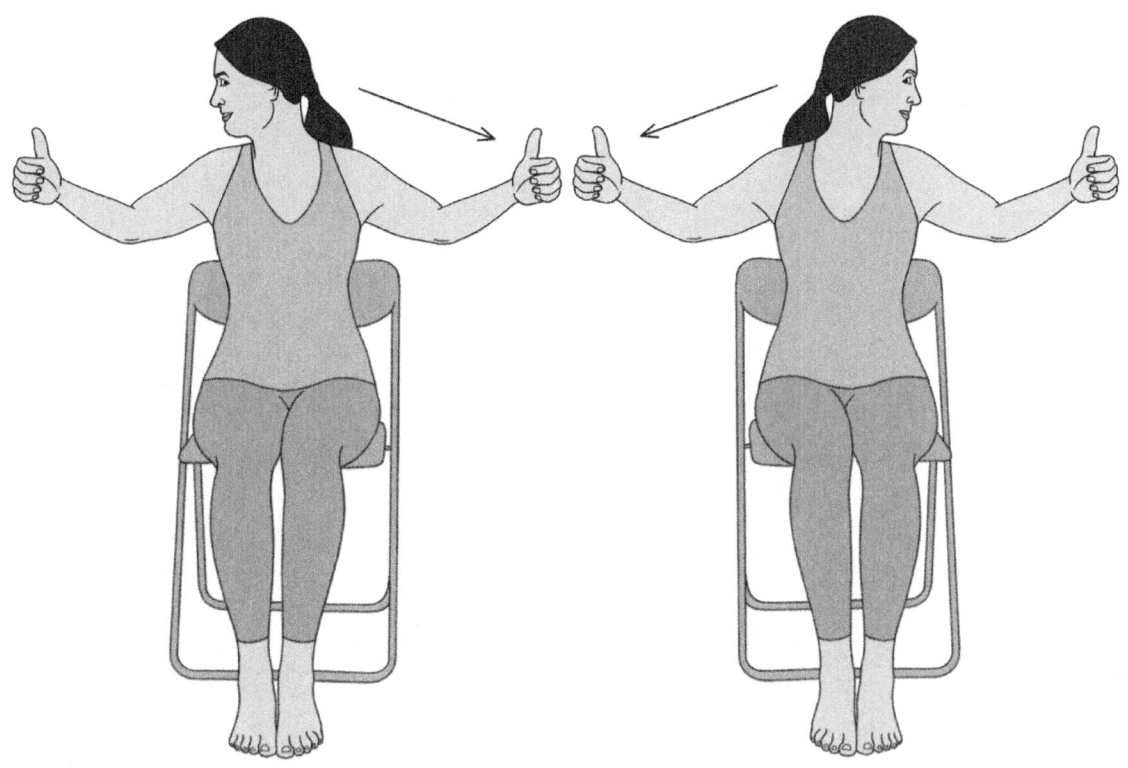

- Sitting in a chair with your back straight, extend your arms outward and stretch them in front of you.
- Turn your head to the right and focus your gaze on your right thumb.
- While keeping your head turned to the right, shift your eyes to the left to focus on your left thumb.
- Repeat this exercise on the other side, turning your head to the left and focusing on your left thumb before shifting your eyes to the right thumb.

This exercise is crucial for controlling the dissociation between head and eye movements.

Arm-Eye coordination

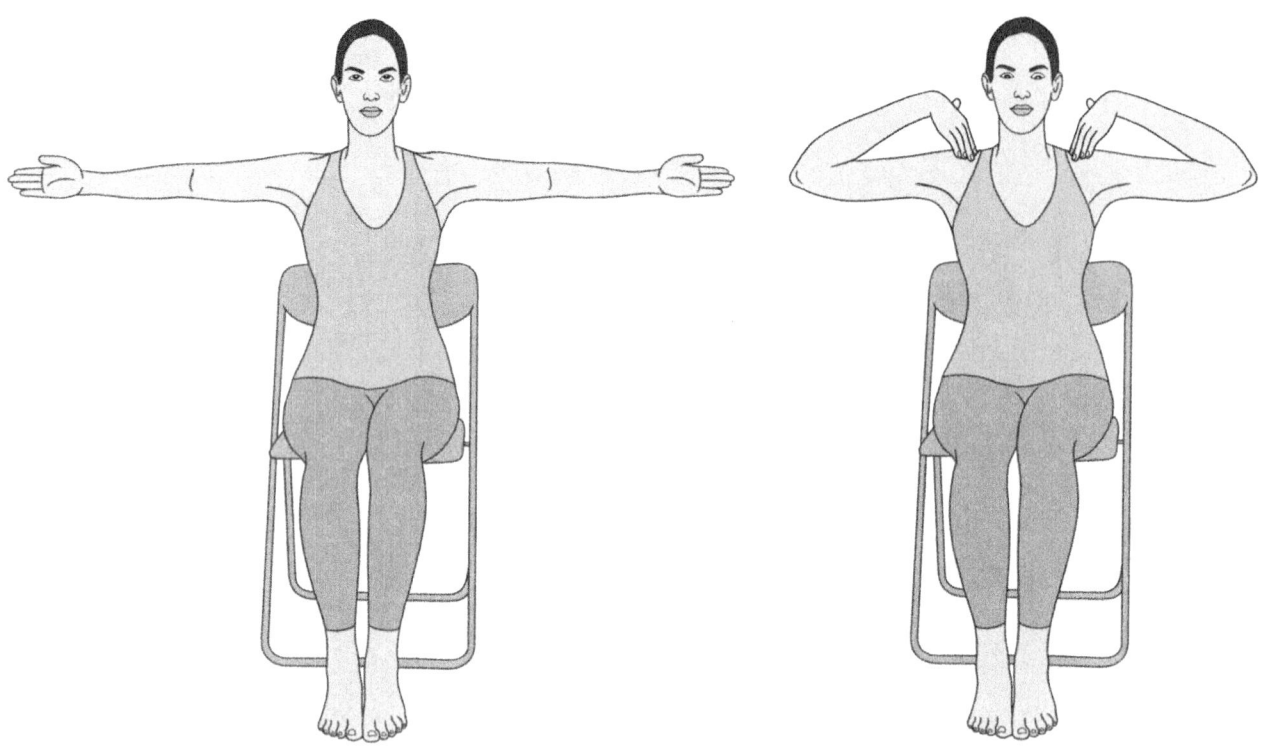

- Begin by sitting with your arms open and your gaze directed upward.
- Fold your arms, reaching to touch your shoulders with your hands, while simultaneously turning your gaze downward.
- Repeat this motion several times at a pace that feels comfortable for you.

Advanced arm-Eye coordination

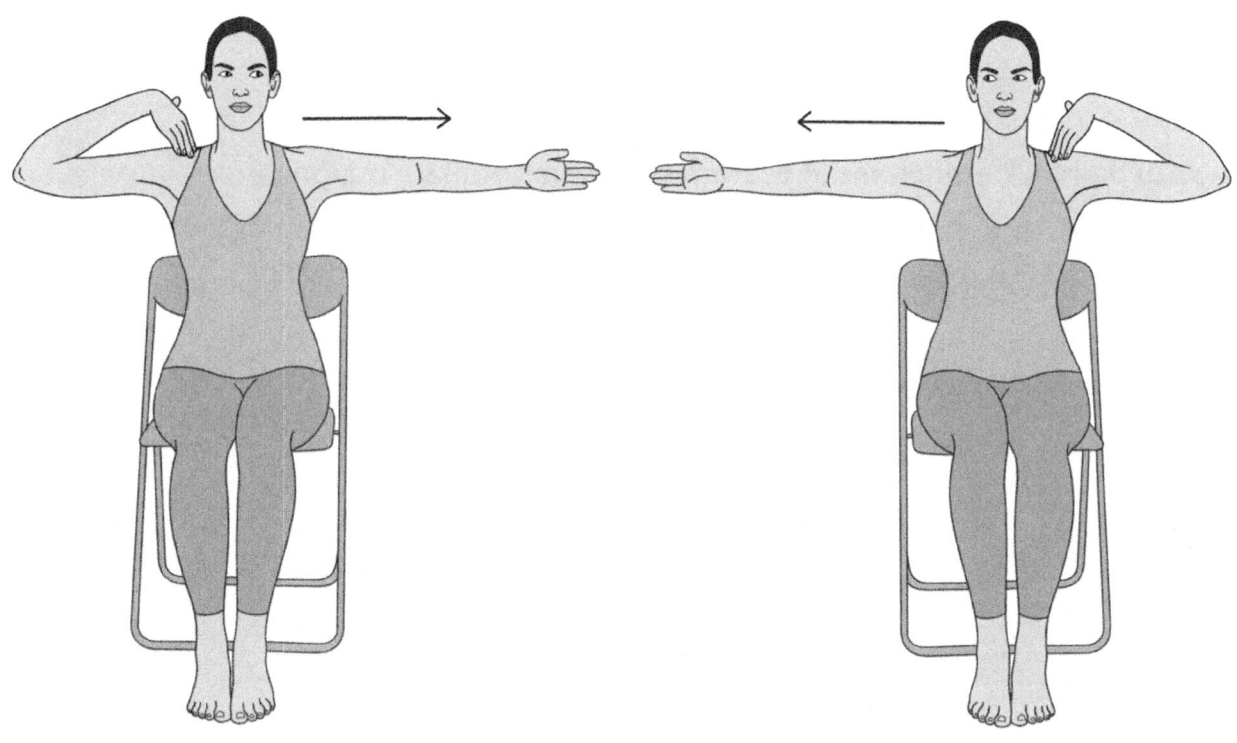

- Sit in a chair with your arms outstretched to the sides.
- Bend your right arm until it touches your right shoulder, while simultaneously turning your gaze to the left towards your hand.
- Return to the starting position with your gaze facing forward.
- Now, bend your left arm until it touches your left shoulder, while turning your gaze to the right towards your hand.
- Repeat this sequence several times to complete the exercise.

SCAN THE QR CODE BELOW to gain access to a comprehensive collection of videos where each balance exercise is broken down step by step and performed by one of my students. This resource will guide you through the exercises, ensuring proper execution and maximizing the benefits of the program.

Plus, you'll unlock a substantial portion of a Revolutionary recipe book.
By integrating these holistic approaches into your lifestyle, you can proactively address balance concerns and cultivate a sense of harmony and vitality.

BALANCE EXERCISES

After dedicating some time to vision exercises, it's crucial to now shift our focus to the next chapter, which explores dynamic balance exercises. While our eyes help us perceive the world, maintaining stability and body control is equally vital for moving confidently.

In this chapter, we'll delve into exercises to improve dynamic balance, helping you stay stable while moving in various ways and on different surfaces. These exercises are accessible to everyone and can bring satisfaction with consistent effort. Additionally, we'll introduce exercises to strengthen your muscles, essential for supporting movements and maintaining posture.

Are you ready for this next step in your journey to better health and fitness?
Let's begin and work towards achieving our balance and strength goals together!

Sit to Stand

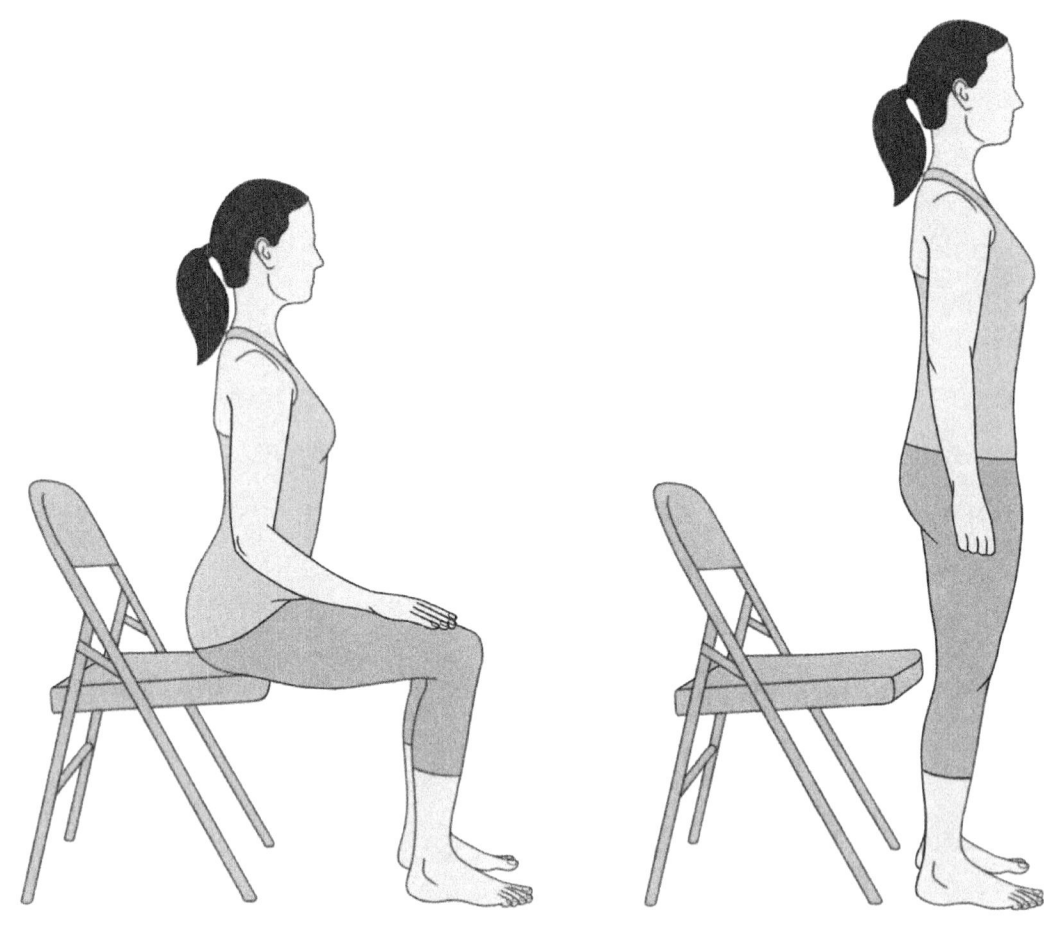

Sit to Stand is a fundamental exercise aimed at improving lower body strength and stability. By transitioning from a seated to a standing position and back again, you engage key muscle groups in the legs while also challenging balance and coordination.

How to do it:

- Sit upright in a sturdy chair with your feet flat on the ground.
- Lean slightly forward to engage your leg muscles.
- Push through your heels to rise from the chair, keeping your back straight.
- Slowly lower yourself back down into the chair, bending your knees and hips as you descend.
- Once seated, reset your posture and repeat the exercise for the desired number of reps.

Benefits:

- Strengthens the muscles in the legs, including the quadriceps, hamstrings, and glutes.
- Improves lower body endurance and functional mobility for activities of daily living.
- Enhances balance and coordination by challenging stability during the transition from sitting to standing.
- Promotes proper posture and alignment, particularly in the spine and hips.

Tip-toe Balance

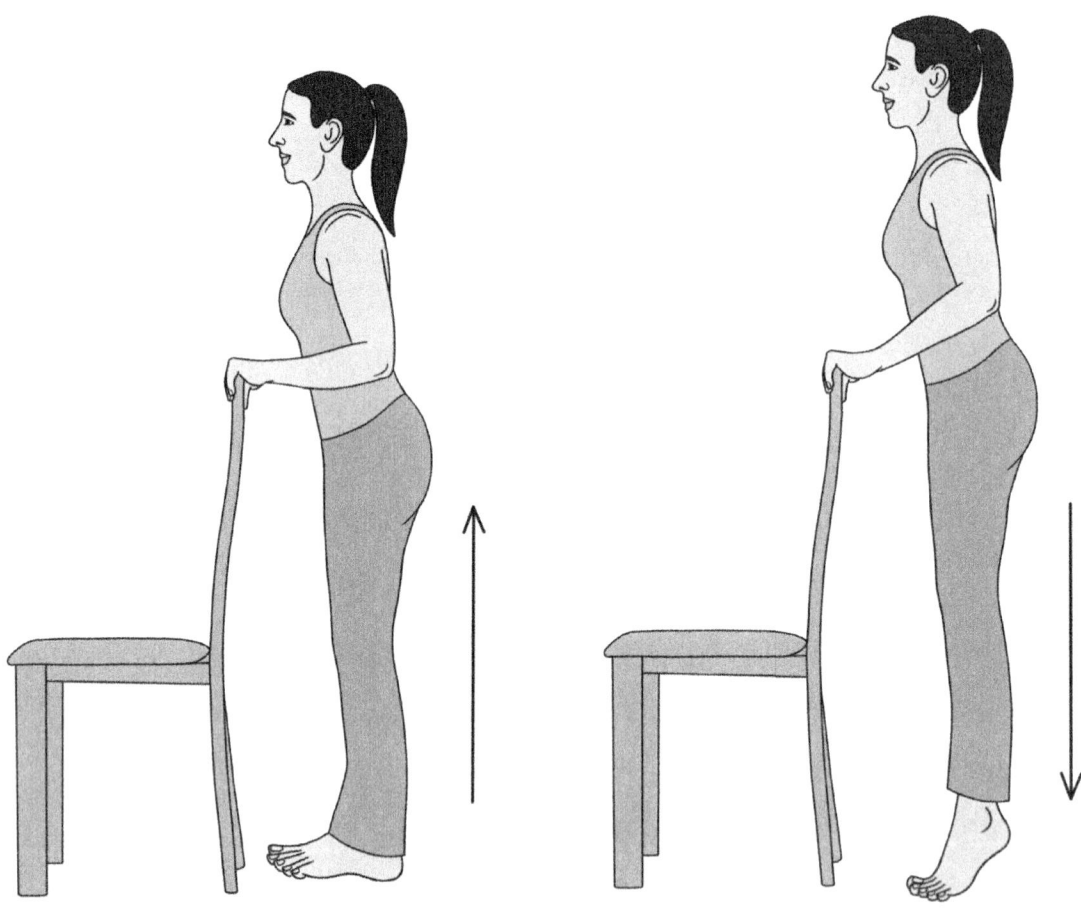

The Tip-toe Balance exercise is designed to improve balance and strengthen the lower body muscles, particularly the calves. Maintaining balance on tiptoes engages various muscle groups, enhancing stability and coordination.

How to do it:

- Stand tall with your spine straight, using a sturdy chair for support by placing your hands on it.
- Lift yourself onto your tiptoes while looking up, ensuring a smooth and controlled movement.
- Hold the position briefly, feeling the engagement of your calf muscles.
- Gently lower your heels back down to the floor, maintaining stability throughout the movement.
- Repeat this motion several times, aiming for a fluid and controlled motion with each repetition.

Benefits:

- Strengthens the lower body muscles, particularly the calves.
- Improves balance and stability.
- Enhances coordination and proprioception.
- Promotes ankle strength and mobility.

Advanced Tip-toe Balance

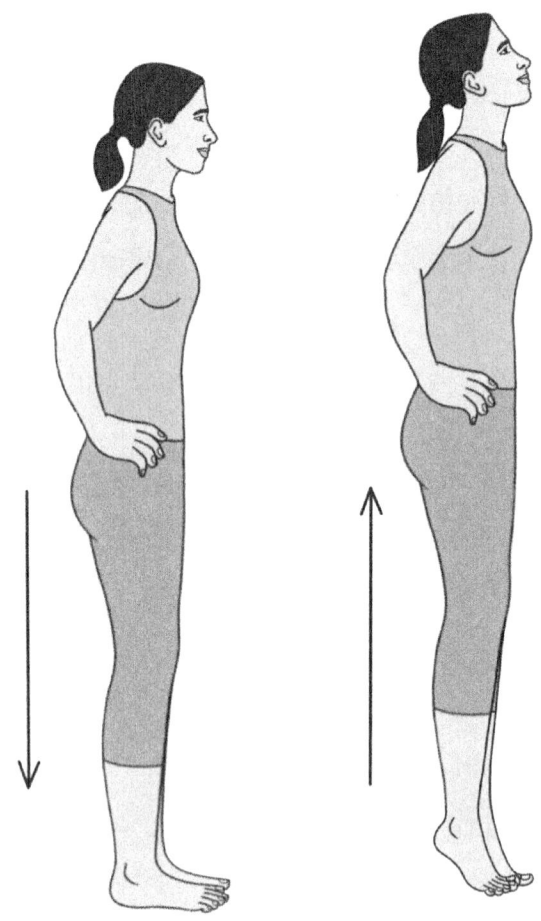

The Advanced Tip-toe Balance exercise presents a heightened challenge compared to the basic tip-toe balance, as it requires maintaining balance without the support of a chair. By lifting onto your tiptoes and gazing upward, you engage your leg muscles more intensively to stabilize your body.

How to do it:

- Stand upright with your feet hip-width apart and your hands resting comfortably by your sides.
- Slowly rise onto your tiptoes, lifting your heels off the floor. Keep your gaze fixed upward to help maintain your balance.
- Hold the lifted position momentarily, focusing on stabilizing your body without leaning forward or backward.
- Lower your heels back down to the floor in a controlled manner, returning to the starting position.
- Repeat the exercise several times, ensuring smooth and controlled movements with each repetition.

Benefits:

- Challenges balance and coordination.
- Strengthens leg muscles, including calves and ankles.
- Enhances overall stability and proprioception.
- Improves ankle joint mobility and flexibility.
- Increases lower body strength and endurance.

Basic Toe Balance

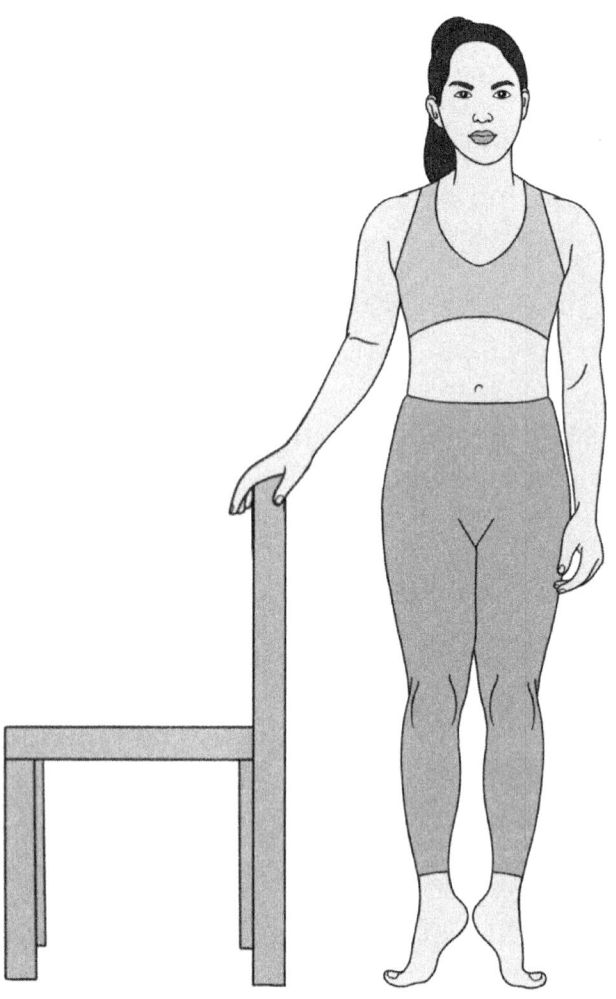

The Basic Toe Balance exercise focuses on enhancing balance and strengthening the lower leg muscles. It serves as a foundational practice for improving stability and control, especially for individuals who may require additional support from a chair or solid surface.

How to do it:

- Begin by standing upright with your feet hip-width apart. If needed, utilize a chair or solid support for assistance.
- Slowly rise onto the tips of your toes, lifting your heels off the ground. Maintain a straight posture with your core engaged.
- Hold the balanced position for a few breaths, focusing on stabilizing your body and maintaining control.
- Lower your heels back to the ground in a controlled manner, returning to the starting position.
- Repeat the exercise several times, aiming for smooth and controlled movements with each repetition.

Benefits:

- Enhances balance and stability.
- Strengthens the muscles in the lower legs, including the calves and ankles.
- Improves ankle joint mobility and flexibility.
- Increases proprioception and body awareness.
- Builds lower body strength and endurance.

Advanced Toe Balance

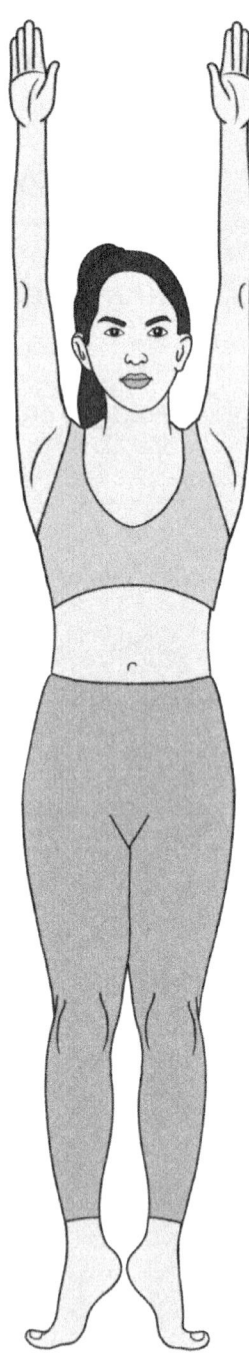

The Advanced Toe Balance exercise is designed to challenge and further develop your balance, requiring increased stability and control compared to the basic version. It involves standing on the tips of your toes while incorporating arm movement and focused visual attention to enhance balance and proprioception.

How to do it:

- Begin by standing tall on the tips of your toes, ensuring proper alignment and engaging your core muscles for stability.
- Raise your arms above your head, extending them upwards with palms facing each other or clasped together.
- Focus your gaze on a specific point in front of you to help maintain balance and concentration.
- Hold the balanced position for a few breaths, maintaining control and stability throughout.
- Slowly lower your heels back to the ground in a controlled manner, returning to the starting position.
- Repeat the exercise several times, aiming for smooth and controlled movements with each repetition.

*Perform this exercise only if you feel confident; otherwise, concentrate on the basic version explained on the previous page.

Benefits:

- Challenges balance and stability at an advanced level.
- Strengthens the muscles of the lower legs, ankles, and core.
- Enhances proprioception and body awareness.
- Improves concentration and focus.
- Promotes overall lower body strength and control.

Toe-Heel Balance

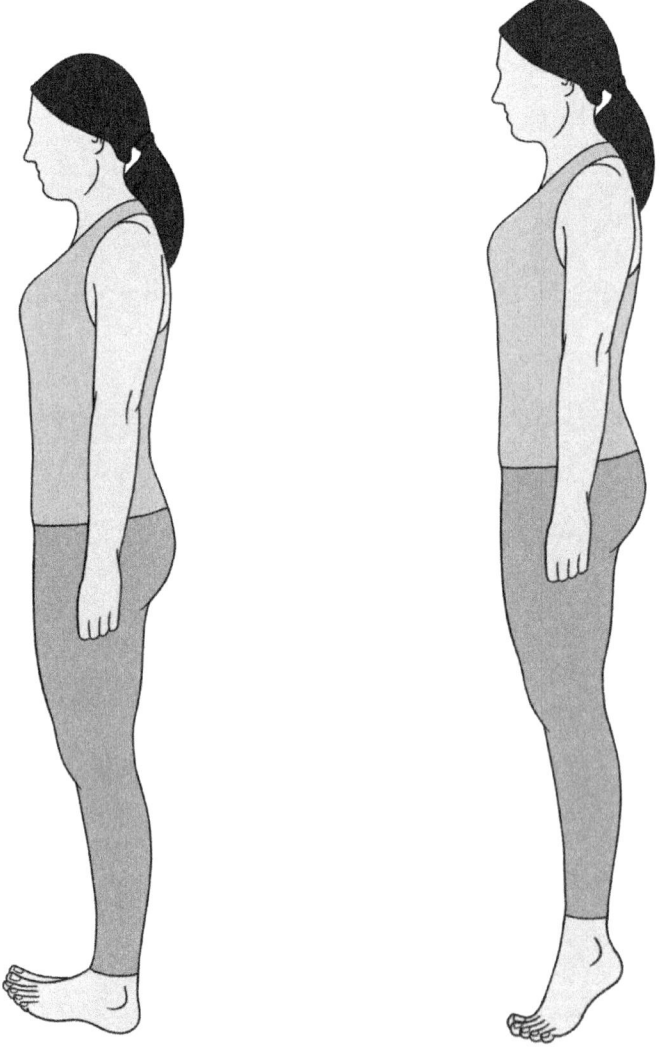

The Toe-Heel Balance exercise is designed to improve balance and proprioception by challenging weight distribution between the toes and heels. It targets the muscles of the feet, ankles, and lower legs, promoting stability and control in various weight-bearing positions.

How to do it:

- Stand upright with your feet hip-width apart, maintaining a straight posture and engaging your core muscles.
- Lift yourself up onto your toes, shifting your weight forward onto the balls of your feet.
- Hold this position momentarily, focusing on maintaining your balance and stability.
- Slowly shift your weight back onto your heels while lifting your toes off the ground as high as possible.
- Hold the heel-raised position briefly, feeling the stretch in your calf muscles.
- Repeat the sequence by shifting back onto your toes, then onto your heels, for several reps.

Benefits:

- Improves balance and stability by challenging weight distribution.
- Strengthens the muscles of the feet, ankles, and lower legs.
- Enhances proprioception and body awareness.
- Increases ankle mobility and flexibility.
- Promotes better posture and alignment.

Tip-toe Walk

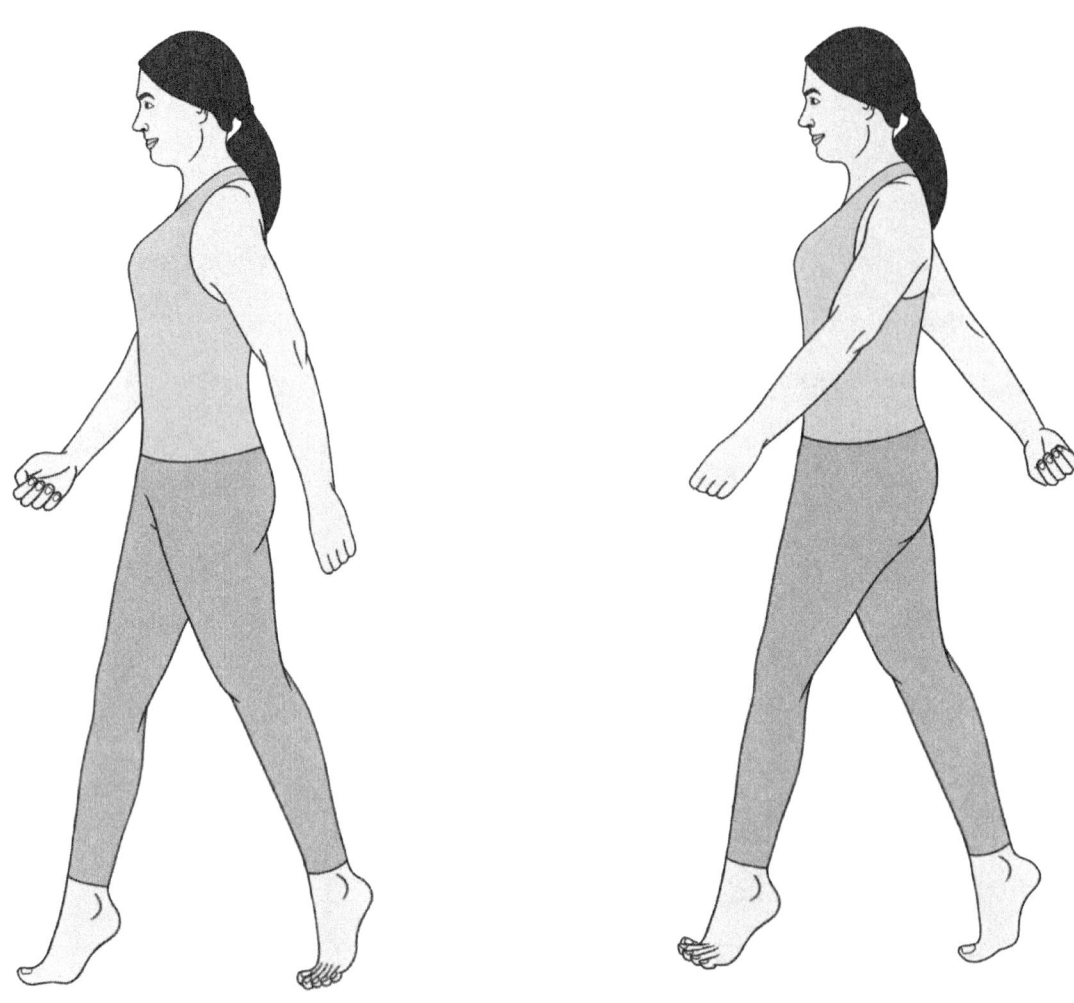

The Tip-Toe Walk exercise challenges balance and strengthens the muscles of the feet, ankles, and lower legs. By walking on the tips of your toes, you engage stabilizing muscles and improve proprioception, enhancing overall stability and control.

How to do it:

- Begin by standing upright, lifting yourself onto the tips of your toes.
- Engage your core muscles to maintain stability and keep your back straight.
- Start walking forward slowly, imagining an invisible line on the floor to guide your steps.
- Take small, controlled steps, placing one foot in front of the other.
- Keep your gaze fixed on a point in front of you to improve balance and focus.
- Continue walking forward for a set distance or time, maintaining balance and control throughout the exercise.

Benefits:

- Strengthens the muscles of the feet, ankles, and lower legs.
- Improves balance, coordination, and proprioception.
- Enhances stability and control during dynamic movements.
- Promotes better posture and alignment.
- Increases ankle mobility and flexibility.

Heel Walk

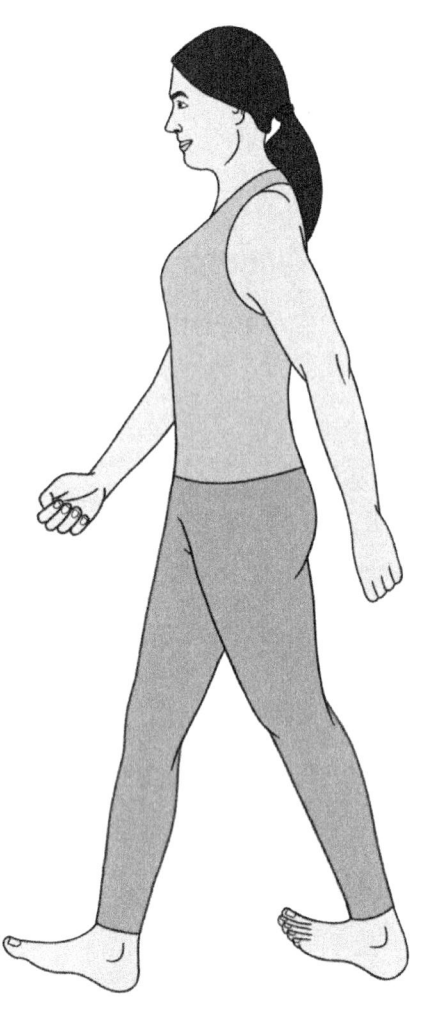 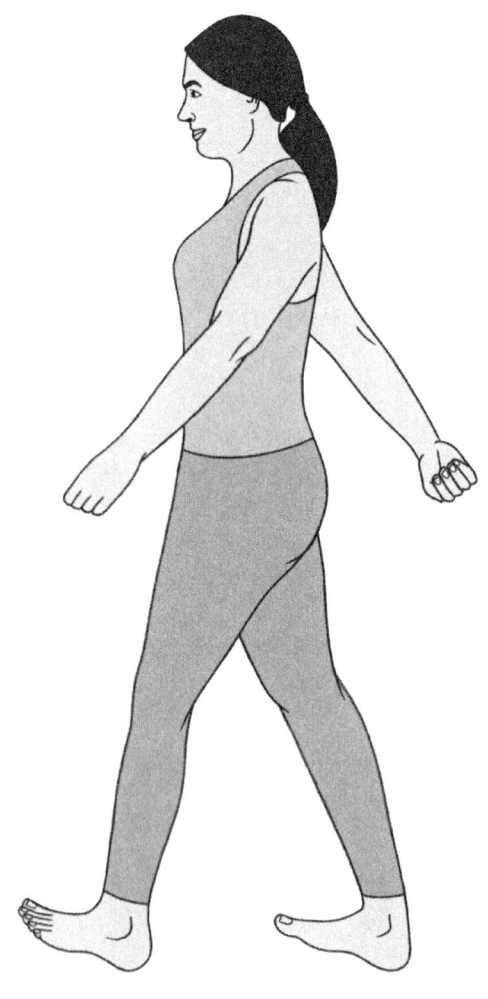

The Heel Walk exercise targets the muscles of the calves, ankles, and feet, providing a unique challenge to balance and stability. By walking on your heels, you engage different muscle groups than during a regular walk, promoting strength and coordination in the lower body.

How to do it:

- Begin by standing upright with your feet hip-width apart.
- Lift your toes off the ground, balancing on your heels.
- Keep your back straight and your gaze forward to maintain proper alignment.
- Start walking forward slowly, placing one heel in front of the other.
- Imagine an invisible line on the floor to guide your steps and maintain a straight path.
- Focus your eyes on a fixed point ahead of you to enhance balance and stability.
- Continue walking forward for a set distance or time, maintaining control and balance throughout the exercise.

Benefits:

- Targets and strengthens the muscles of the calves, ankles, and feet.
- Improves balance, stability, and proprioception.
- Enhances ankle mobility and flexibility.
- Promotes proper posture and alignment.
- Provides a unique challenge to the lower body muscles.

Baby Steps

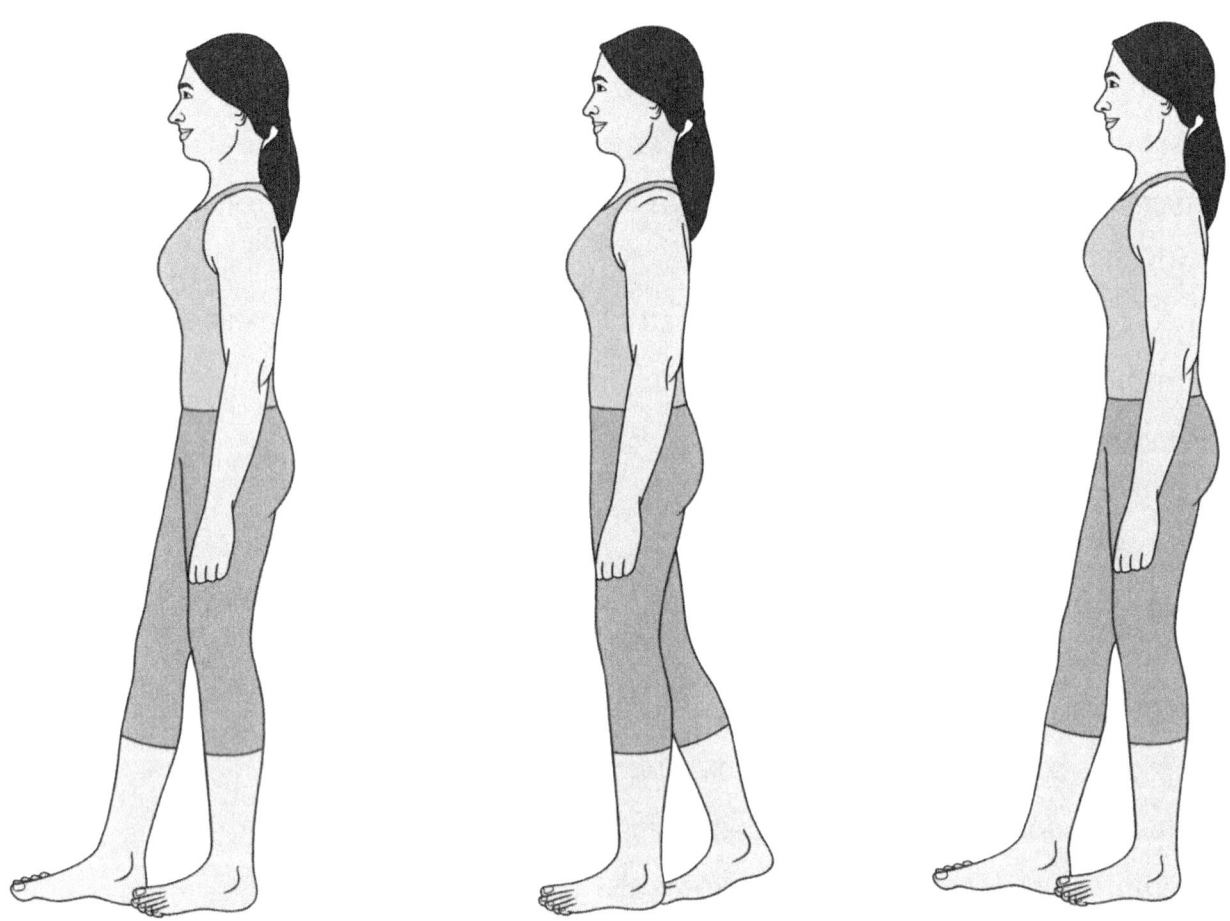

The Baby Steps exercise involves taking small, deliberate steps forward, emphasizing balance and coordination. By maintaining proper alignment and focus, you can enhance your stability and control while moving.

How to do it:

- Stand upright with your feet together, maintaining a straight posture.
- Take a small step forward with your right foot, placing it directly in front of your left foot.
- Bring your left foot forward, aligning it with your right foot.
- Continue taking small steps forward, ensuring that each foot lands directly in front of the other, without any space between them.
- Imagine following an imaginary line on the floor to guide your steps and maintain proper alignment.
- Keep your gaze forward and focus on a fixed point in front of you to improve balance and stability.
- Repeat the movement for a set distance or time, maintaining control and balance throughout the exercise.

Benefits:

- Enhances balance and coordination.
- Strengthens lower body muscles, including the calves, thighs, and ankles.
- Improves proprioception and spatial awareness.
- Promotes proper posture and alignment.
- Provides a controlled and deliberate movement pattern for stability training.

March Steps

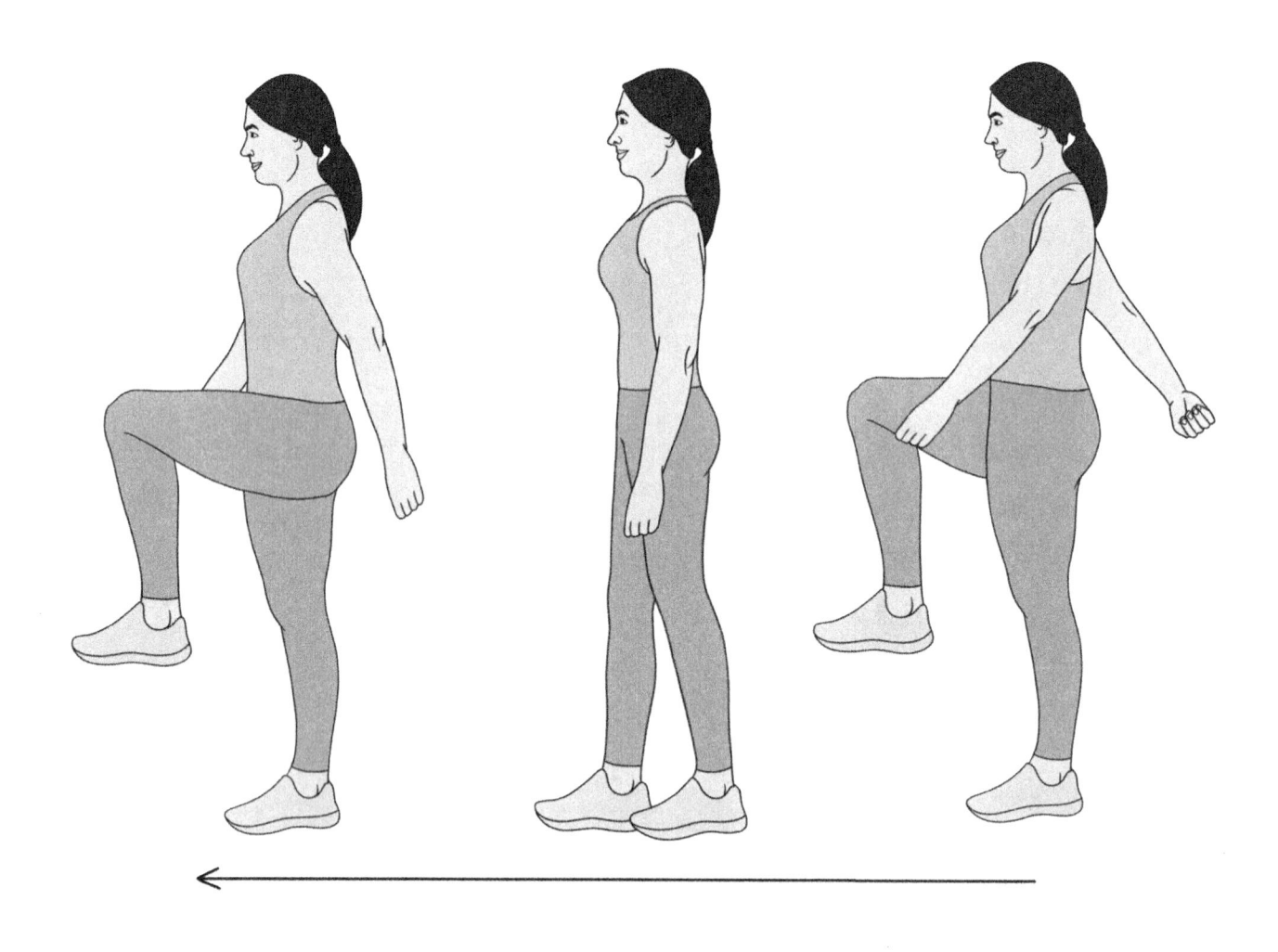

March Steps is a dynamic exercise that combines walking with intentional knee lifts to improve balance, strength, and coordination. By focusing on lifting the knees high and maintaining balance throughout the movement, you can enhance lower body stability and mobility.

How to do it:

- Begin by standing tall with your feet together and your arms relaxed at your sides.
- Imagine an imaginary line on the ground in front of you as your path for walking.
- Lift your right knee up towards your chest, aiming to bring it parallel to the floor.
- Place your right foot down gently on the imaginary line, maintaining your balance.
- As you step forward with your right foot, simultaneously lift your left knee towards your chest in a marching motion.
- Continue alternating between lifting the knees of each leg as you walk forward along the imaginary line.
- Focus on maintaining an upright posture, engaging your core muscles for stability, and keeping a steady pace.
- Aim to lift your knees as high as possible with each step while maintaining control and balance.

Benefits:

- Improves balance and coordination by challenging stability with each step.
- Strengthens the lower body muscles, including the quadriceps, hamstrings, and glutes.
- Enhances mobility and flexibility in the hips and knees.
- Promotes proper gait mechanics and alignment.
- Provides a cardiovascular workout while engaging multiple muscle groups.

Side Leg Raise

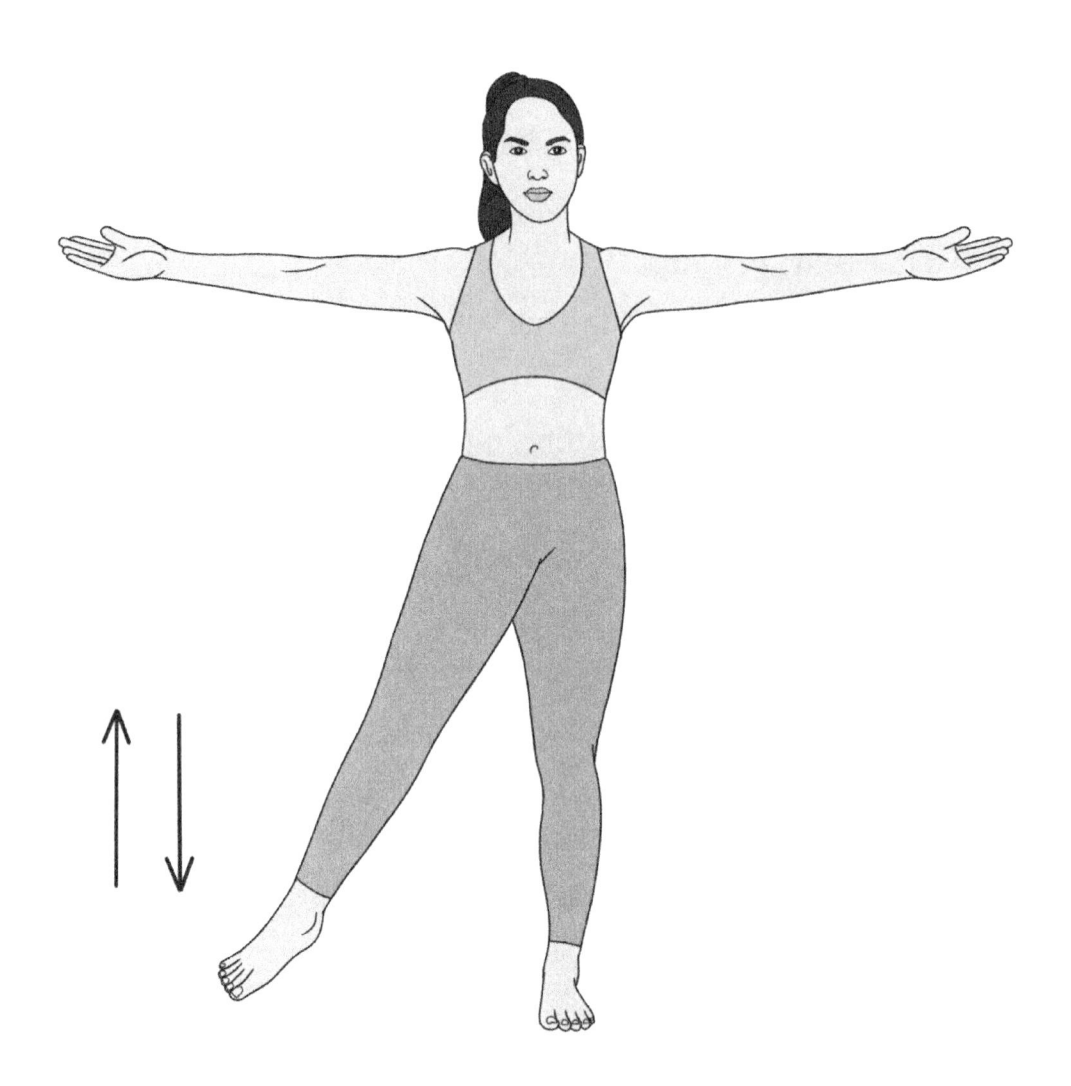

The side leg raise exercise targets the muscles of the hips and outer thighs, helping to improve hip stability and strengthen the muscles responsible for lateral movement. It's a great exercise for enhancing overall lower body strength and stability.

How to do it:

- Begin by standing upright with your feet hip-width apart and your arms extended straight out to the sides for balance.
- Shift your weight slightly onto your right leg.
- Point your left foot out to the side, keeping your leg straight.
- Engage your outer thigh muscles and lift your left leg out to the side as high as comfortable.
- Slowly lower your left leg back down to the starting position.
- Repeat the same movement with your right leg.
- Continue alternating between raising and lowering each leg while keeping your arms extended straight out to the sides.

Benefits:

- Strengthens the muscles of the hips, outer thighs, and glutes.
- Improves hip stability and balance.
- Enhances overall lower body strength.
- Helps in toning and shaping the legs.
- Can contribute to better functional movement and mobility in daily activities.

Leg Lift

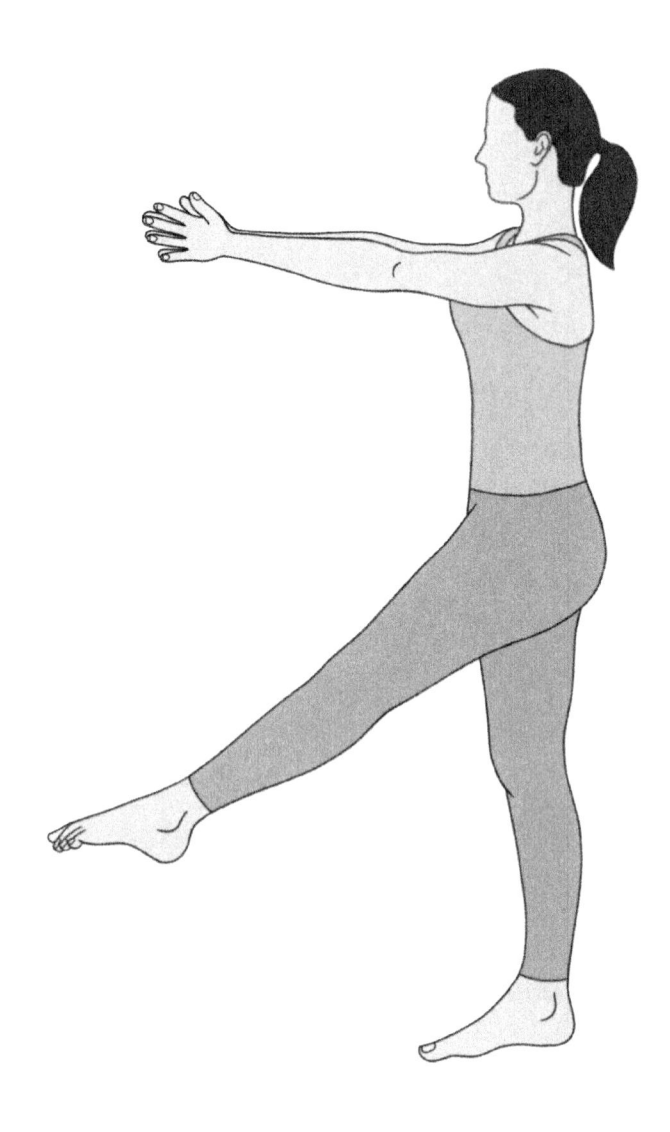

The leg lift exercise targets the muscles of the thighs, hips, and core, helping to improve lower body strength, stability, and balance. It's an effective exercise for toning the legs and enhancing overall mobility.

How to do it:

- Stand upright with your feet hip-width apart and your arms extended straight in front of you, palms facing each other, and fingers spread apart. Keep your gaze forward.
- Lift your right leg in front of you, raising it as high as you can while maintaining control and stability.
- Hold this position for a few breaths, focusing on maintaining your balance and engaging your core muscles.
- Slowly lower your right leg back to the ground.
- Repeat the exercise with your left leg, lifting it in front of you and holding the position for a few breaths.
- Continue alternating legs for several reps to complete the exercise.

Benefits:

- Strengthens the muscles of the thighs, hips, and core.
- Improves lower body stability and balance.
- Helps in toning and shaping the legs.
- Enhances overall mobility and functional movement.

Advanced Leg Lift

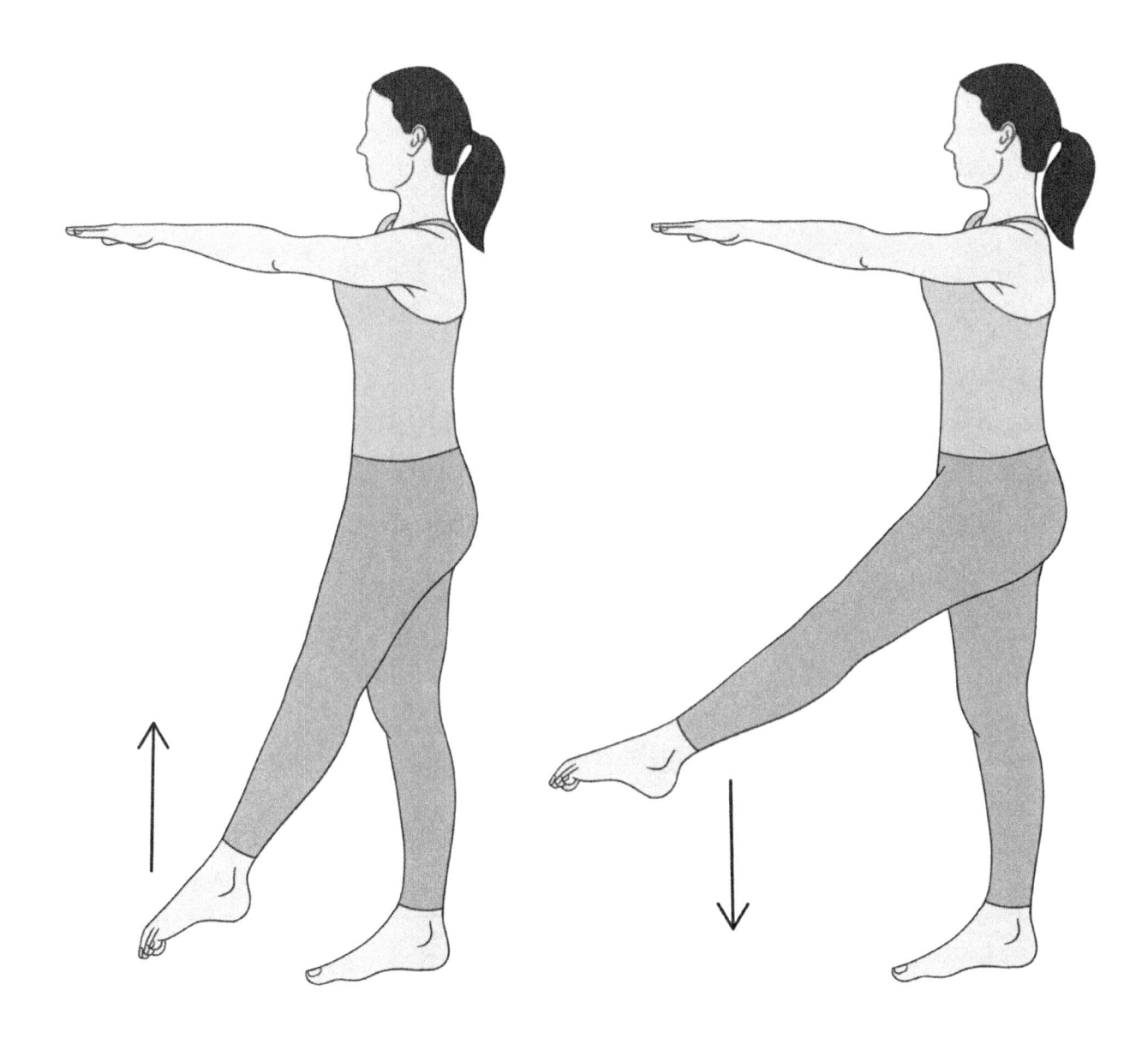

The advanced leg lift exercise is a progression from the basic leg lift, focusing on further challenging the muscles of the legs, hips, and core. It requires greater balance, stability, and control to perform effectively.

How to do it:

- Stand upright with your feet hip-width apart and your arms extended straight in front of you.
- Lift your left leg off the ground, keeping it straight and the toes pointed downward.
- Hold the lifted position briefly, engaging your core muscles for stability.
- Slowly lower your left leg back down to the ground.
- Repeat the same movement with your right leg, lifting it off the ground while keeping it straight and the toes pointed downward.
- Alternate between lifting and lowering each leg for several reps, maintaining control and stability throughout the exercise.

Benefits:

- Strengthens the muscles of the legs, hips, and core.
- Improves balance, stability, and proprioception.
- Challenges coordination and control.
- Enhances lower body strength and functional mobility.

Single-Leg Balance

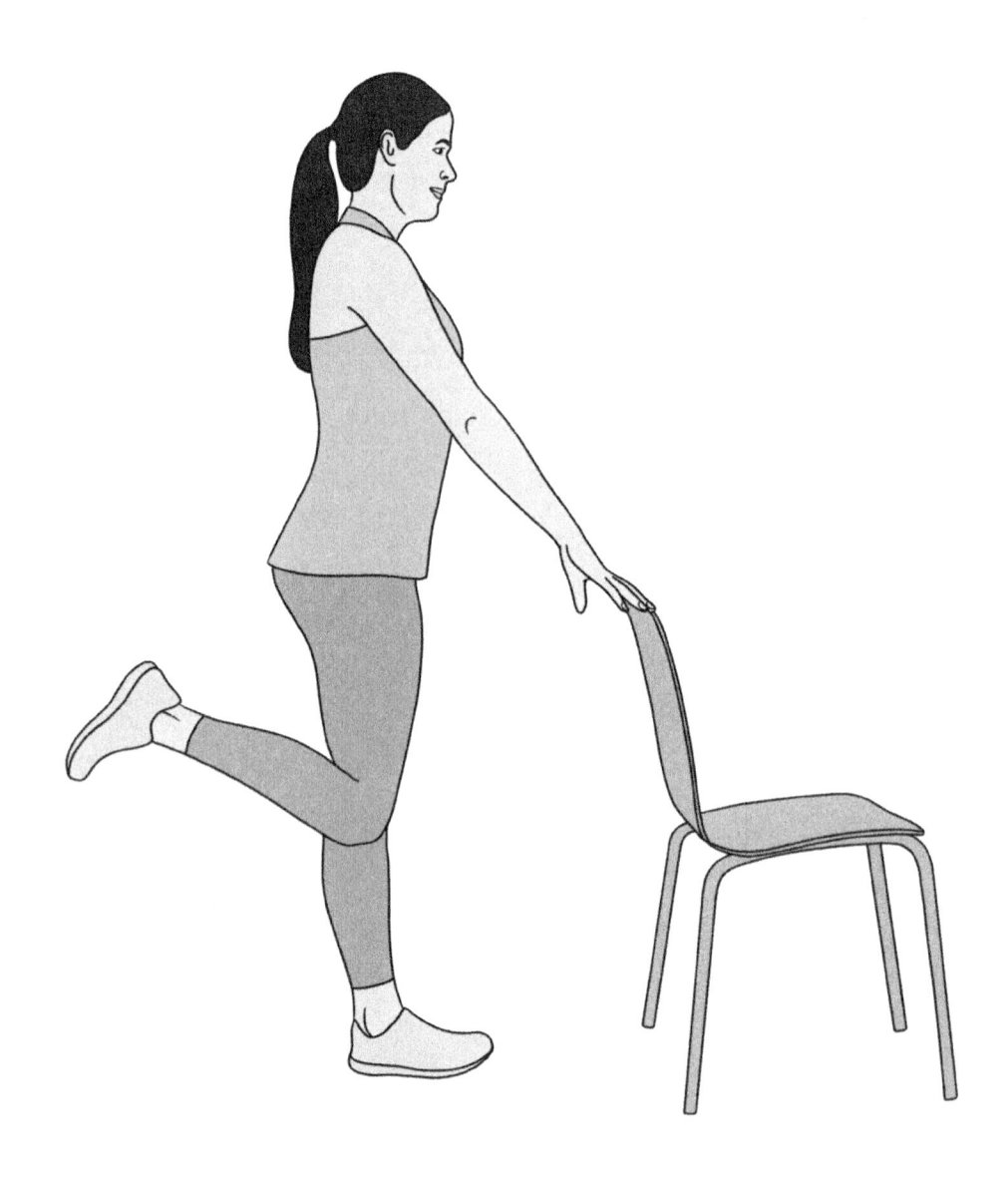

The single-leg balance exercise is designed to improve balance, stability, and proprioception. By challenging the body to maintain equilibrium on one leg, this exercise strengthens the muscles of the lower body and enhances overall stability.

How to do it:

- Begin by standing upright with your back straight, using a chair or solid support for assistance if needed.
- Extend your right leg backward, lifting it off the ground while keeping your balance with the support of the chair.
- Strive to maintain this balanced position for as long as you comfortably can, focusing on stability and control.
- Slowly lower your right leg back to the starting position, maintaining control throughout the movement.
- Repeat the process with your left leg, ensuring to maintain stability with the support of the chair or solid object.
- Engage your core muscles throughout the exercise to help stabilize your body and maintain balance.
- Continue alternating between lifting your right and left legs, focusing on maintaining balance and control with each repetition.

Benefits:

- Improves balance and stability.
- Strengthens the muscles of the lower body, including the hips, thighs, and calves.
- Enhances proprioception and body awareness.
- Helps prevent falls and injuries by improving stability and coordination.
- Engages the core muscles for added support and stability during movement.

Advanced Single-Leg Balance

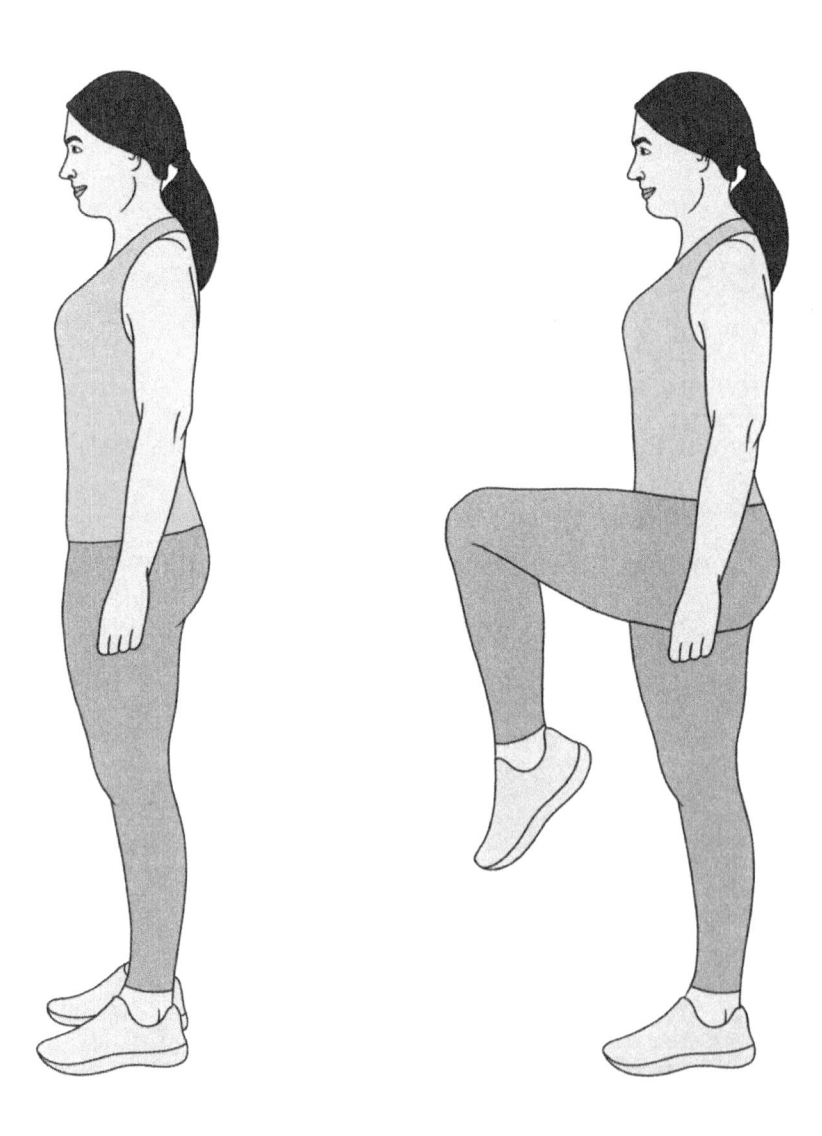

The advanced single-leg balance exercise builds upon the basic single-leg balance by increasing the challenge to stability and proprioception. By lifting one leg off the ground and maintaining balance without support, this exercise further strengthens the muscles of the lower body and core while enhancing overall stability and coordination.

How to do it:

- Stand tall with your arms relaxed at your sides and maintain a forward gaze, focusing on a fixed point for stability.
- Lift one leg off the ground while engaging your abdominal muscles to stabilize your body and maintain balance.
- Take a deep breath in, exhale, and then switch to lift the other leg off the ground.
- Continue alternating legs while focusing on maintaining steady breathing and balance throughout the exercise.
- Keep your movements slow and controlled, avoiding any sudden jerks or shifts in weight.
- Focus on maintaining proper posture, with your shoulders back and your core engaged to support your spine.
- Use your arms for balance as needed, but aim to rely primarily on the strength and stability of your lower body and core muscles.

Benefits:

- Increases the challenge to stability and proprioception.
- Strengthens the muscles of the lower body, including the hips, thighs, and calves.
- Engages the core muscles to stabilize the body and maintain balance.
- Improves overall stability and coordination.
- Enhances body awareness and mindfulness.

Back Leg Extensions

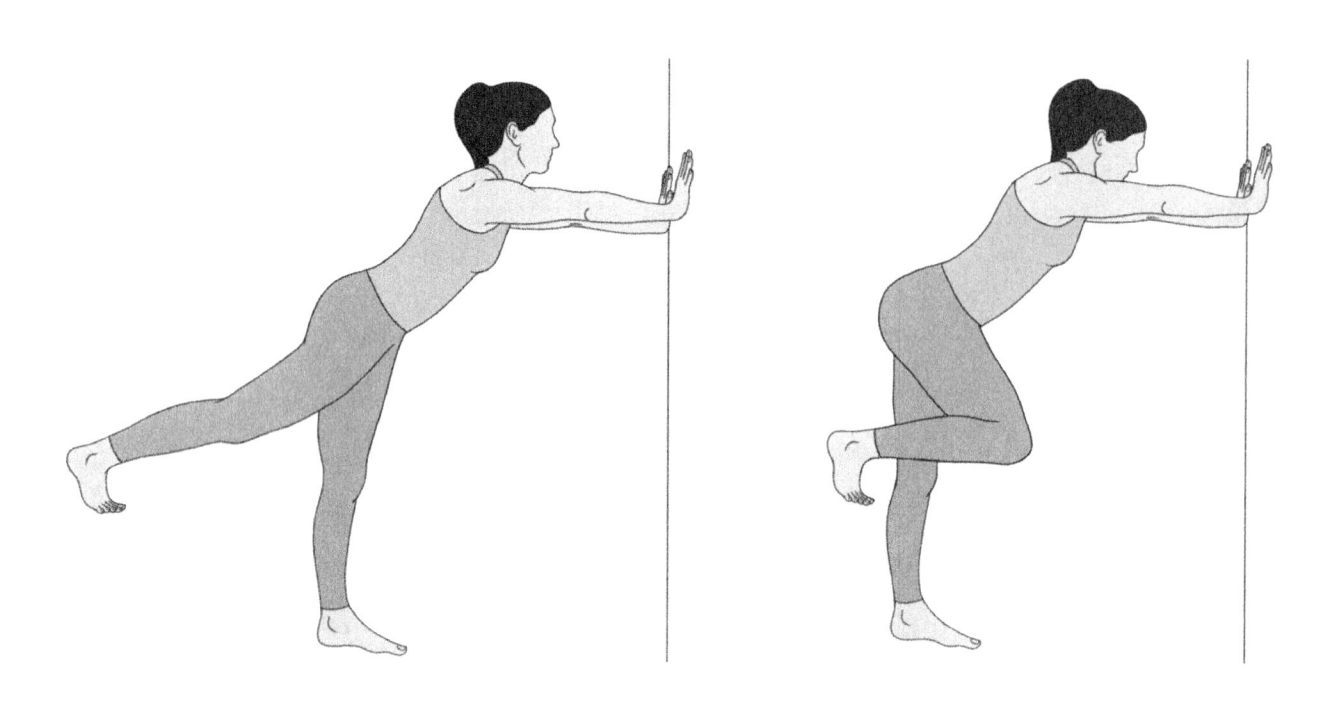

Back leg extensions are an effective exercise for strengthening the muscles of the lower body, particularly the glutes and hamstrings. By extending one leg behind you while standing, you engage these muscles to improve strength, stability, and balance.

How to do it:

- Stand upright with your back against a wall, ensuring proper posture with your shoulders back and your spine aligned.
- Bend your right leg at the knee while keeping your back straight and your foot flat on the ground.
- Slowly extend your right leg behind you, focusing on keeping it straight and taut.
- Contract your gluteus (buttock muscles) as you extend your leg, feeling the muscles engage.
- Bring your right leg back towards your chest, bending at the knee, while engaging your abdominal muscles to stabilize your body.
- Remember to maintain regular breathing throughout the exercise. Inhale as you extend your leg backward and exhale as you pull your leg back towards your chest.

Benefits:

- Strengthens lower body muscles.
- Improves stability and balance.
- Enhances lower body strength for daily activities.
- Helps prevent injuries by strengthening supporting muscles.
- Promotes better posture and alignment.

Knee Flex and Lift

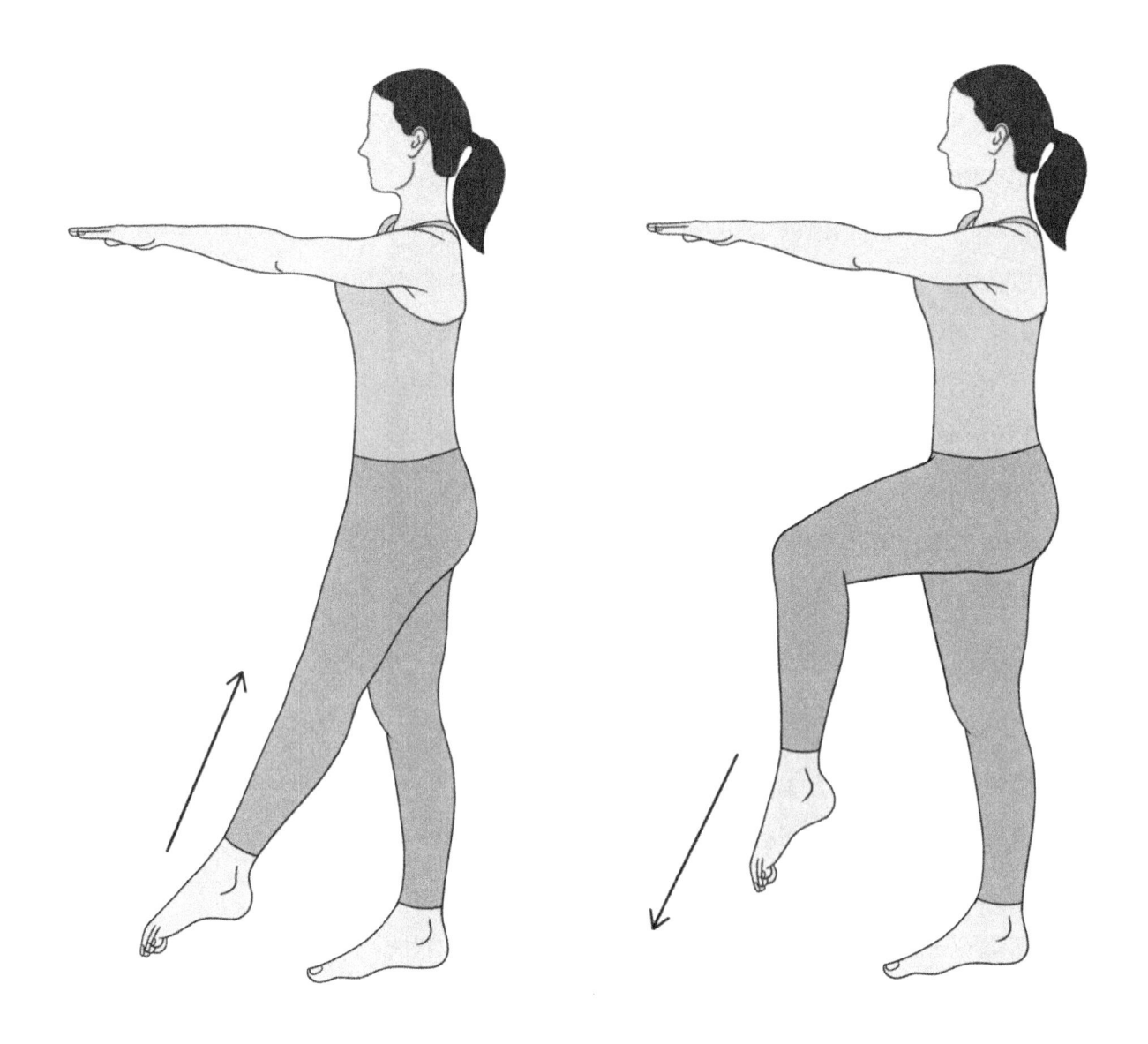

The Knee Flex and Lift exercise targets the quadriceps and aims to enhance knee flexibility and leg strength. This exercise helps improve balance, stability, and overall lower body control.

How to do it:

- Stand tall with a forward gaze, keeping your back straight and arms extended in front of you.
- Lift your left leg in front of you, then bend the knee while pointing your toes downward as you raise it.
- Adjust reps according to your comfort level and ability.
- Repeat the exercise with your other leg, ensuring the same range of motion and control.

Benefits:

- Strengthens quadriceps muscles for improved knee stability and support.
- Enhances flexibility in the knees, promoting better range of motion.
- Improves balance and coordination by engaging core muscles.
- Helps develop leg strength essential for daily activities like walking and standing.

Toe-to-Knee Chair Assisted

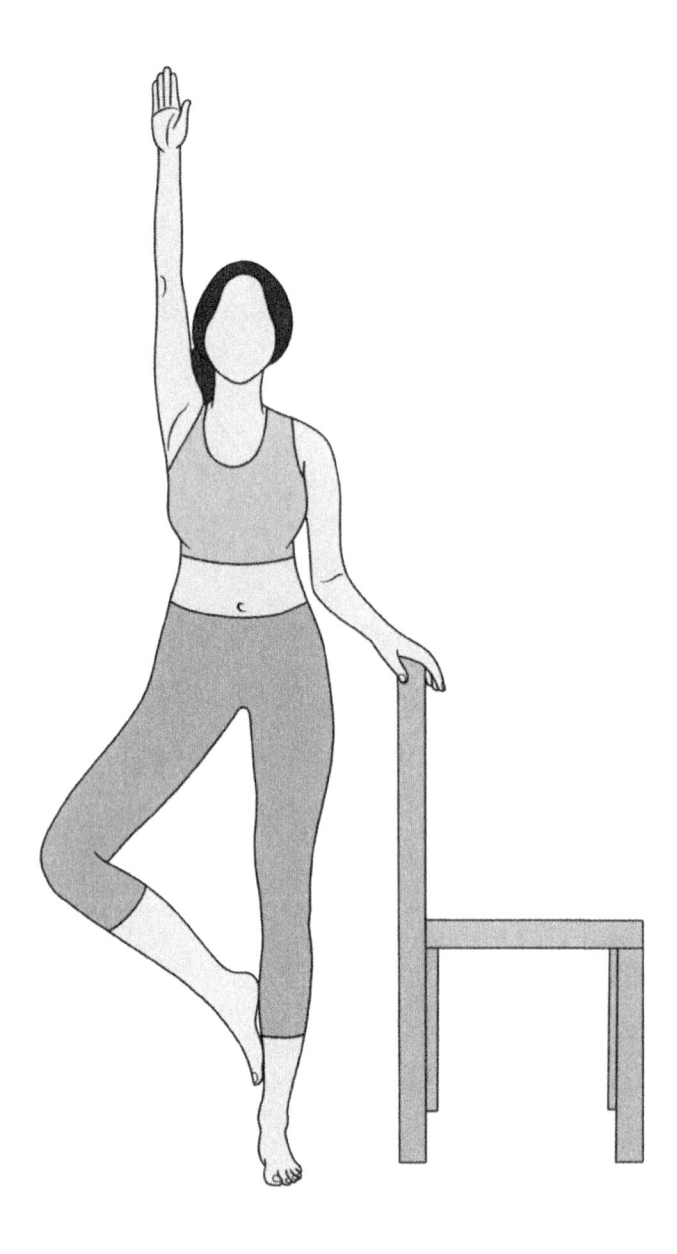

The Toe-to-Knee Chair Assisted exercise is designed to improve balance and stability while strengthening the legs and back. By utilizing a sturdy chair for support, this exercise offers a safe way to enhance lower body strength and coordination.

How to do it:

- Stand next to a sturdy chair, using it for support.
- Lift your right arm while maintaining a straight gaze ahead.
- Raise your right foot and place the sole against the side of your left knee at knee height.
- Take deep breaths and hold the position for as long as you can safely manage, ensuring your back remains straight and your left leg muscles are engaged.
- Repeat the exercise on your left side.

Benefits:

- Strengthens leg muscles, particularly the quadriceps and calves.
- Improves balance and stability by engaging core muscles.
- Enhances coordination between upper and lower body.
- Promotes better posture and spinal alignment.
- Increases body awareness and control.

Ankle Point and Flex

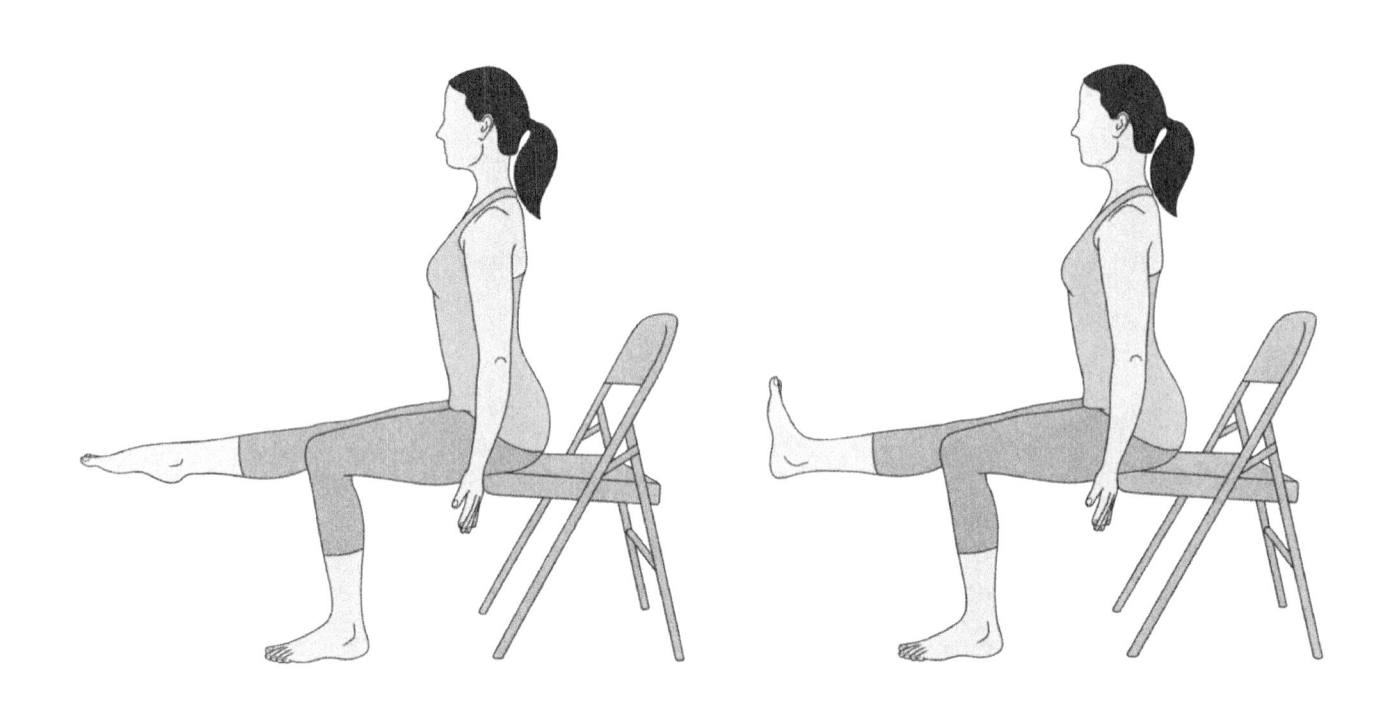

The Ankle Point and Flex exercise targets ankle flexibility and strength while seated in a chair. By alternating between pointing and flexing the ankles, this exercise helps improve range of motion and mobility in the lower legs.

How to do it:

- Start by standing upright with your feet hip-width apart and your arms relaxed at your sides.
- Bend your right leg at the knee, bringing your foot up toward your buttocks while maintaining balance on your left leg.
- Hold the position for as long as possible, focusing on keeping your body stable.
- Switch to your left leg and repeat the exercise, bringing your left foot up toward your buttocks while balancing on your right leg.

If needed, consider using a nearby support such as a chair or wall for stability.

Benefits:

- Improves balance and stability in the lower body.
- Strengthens the muscles of the legs and core.
- Enhances proprioception, or the body's awareness of its position in space.
- Helps prevent falls by increasing stability and coordination.
- Can be easily modified to accommodate different fitness levels and abilities.

Advanced Leg Hold Balance

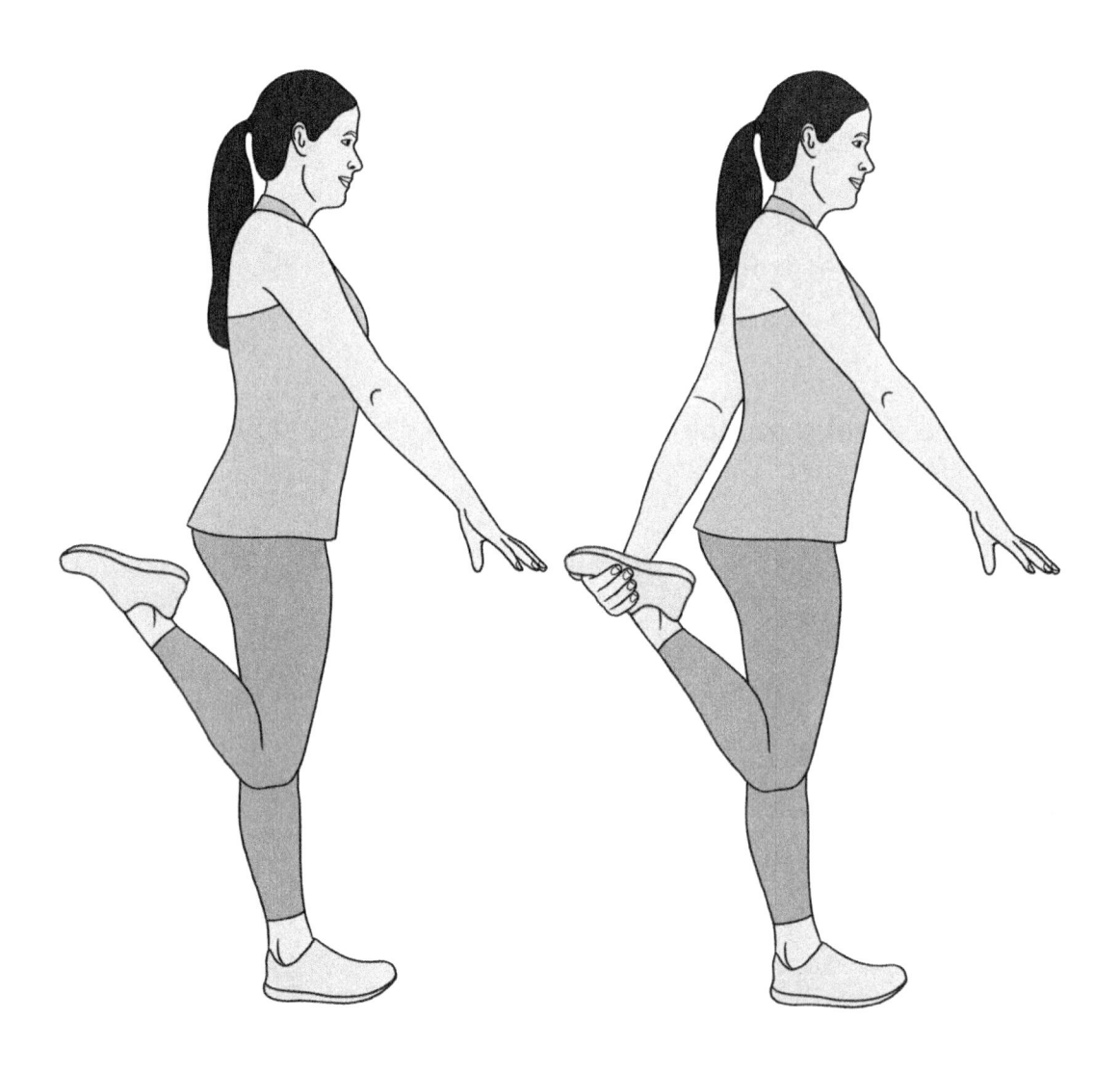

The Advanced Leg Hold Balance exercise is designed to challenge your balance and stability further by incorporating a dynamic movement pattern. This exercise targets the muscles of the lower body and core while also improving proprioception and coordination.

How to do it:

- Start by standing upright with your feet hip-width apart and your arms relaxed at your sides.
- Bend your right leg and reach across your body with your left hand to grasp your right foot.
- Hold this position for as long as possible while engaging your core muscles and focusing on stability.
- Switch sides and repeat the exercise, bending your left leg and reaching across your body with your right hand to grasp your left foot.
- Gradually increase the duration of each hold as your balance improves, aiming to maintain stability for longer periods.

If needed, consider using a nearby support such as a chair or wall for stability.

Benefits:

- Challenges balance and stability in a dynamic movement pattern.
- Strengthens the muscles of the legs, core, and upper body.
- Improves proprioception and coordination by engaging multiple muscle groups simultaneously.
- Enhances overall body awareness and control.
- Can be adapted to suit various fitness levels and abilities, making it accessible to a wide range of individuals.

Dynamic Lunge

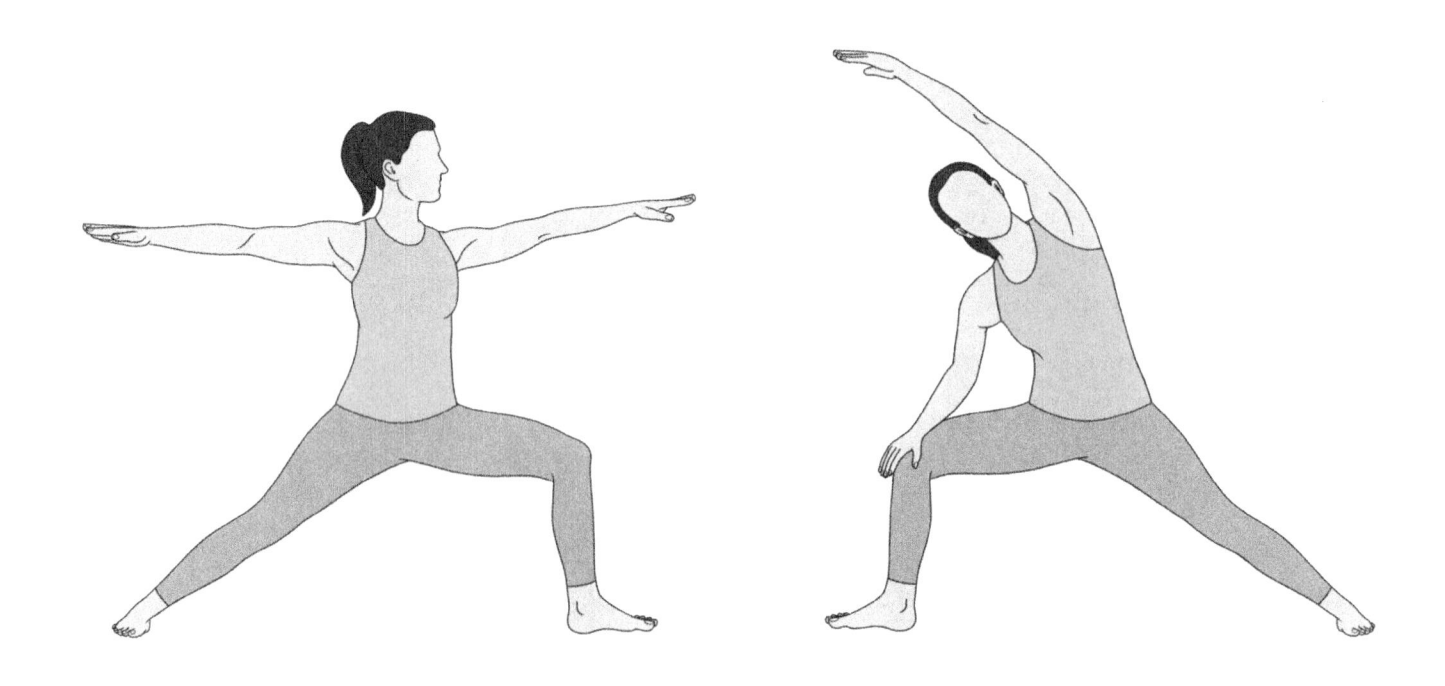

The Dynamic Lunge exercise is a compound movement that targets multiple muscle groups in the lower body while also engaging the core and upper body. By incorporating dynamic movements into the lunge, this exercise enhances balance, coordination, and strength.

How to do it:

- Start in a standing position with your legs spread wide apart and your arms extended horizontally at shoulder height.
- Perform a lunge to the right side by bending your right leg at the knee while keeping your left leg straight and simultaneously raising your right arm above your head.
- At the same time, lower your left arm to rest on your left knee for support.
- Return to the starting position by pushing off your right foot and straightening your right leg, bringing your arms back to the horizontal position.
- Repeat the lunge on the opposite side by bending your left leg and raising your left arm above your head while lowering your right arm to rest on your right knee.

Benefits:

- Targets multiple muscle groups in the lower body, including the quadriceps, hamstrings, glutes, and calves.
- Engages the core muscles for stability and balance.
- Improves coordination and proprioception through dynamic movement patterns.
- Enhances functional strength and mobility, particularly in activities that involve unilateral movements or changes in direction.
- Provides a cardiovascular challenge when performed at a moderate to high intensity, contributing to overall fitness and endurance.

28-DAY PLAN

As you embark on this journey through balance exercises, know that you're not alone. Over the next 28 days, we'll walk together, step by step, towards a stronger and more confident you.

This carefully structured program is tailored for seniors like you, with the aim of bringing remarkable improvements with just a few minutes of dedication each day. Imagine investing a small portion of your time into these exercises and witnessing the profound changes they can bring into your life.

Throughout this journey, these simple yet powerful exercises will become an integral part of your daily routine. They are not just movements; they are tools to help you regain your balance, strength, and confidence. With each passing day, you'll feel steadier and more grounded, reclaiming the confidence you thought you'd lost.

Let this program be your guiding light, a beacon of hope that leads you towards a brighter tomorrow. As we progress together, observe the small victories and celebrate the progress you make. Whether it's feeling more stable on your feet or gaining newfound confidence in your abilities, know that each day brings you closer to a better, more balanced version of yourself.

Visual Warm-Up

At the start of each day in this 28-day plan, we'll begin with what we like to call the "Visual Warm-Up". During this time, we'll engage in a series of eye-focused exercises designed to enhance our visual acuity and awareness.

The Visual Warm-Up, as discussed in the early pages of the book, consists of several key components:

- Ocular Training
- Peripheral Ocular Focus
- Ocular Dissociation
- Arm-Eye Coordination
- Advanced Arm-Eye Coordination

In the following page, we will discuss the Improving Awareness Exercise, which serves as the conclusion to the Visual Warm-Up. This exercise is essential for enhancing our awareness of the environment around us. After completing the Visual Warm-Up, we can then proceed to the balance exercises for the day.

Improving Awareness Exercise

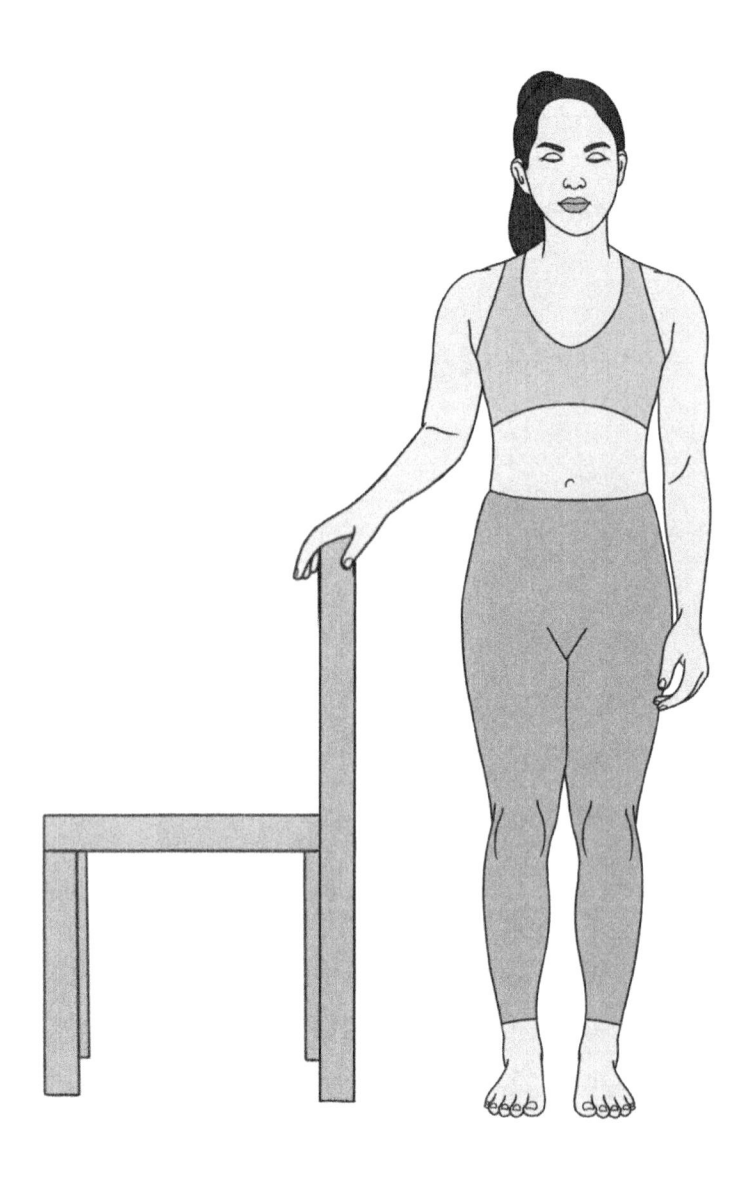

The Improving Awareness Exercise is designed to enhance mindfulness and sensory perception by connecting with the environment around you. By engaging in this exercise, you'll sharpen your awareness of your surroundings and cultivate a deeper sense of presence.

How to do it:

- Begin by standing next to a sturdy chair to provide support for balance.
- Close your eyes and take three deep breaths, allowing yourself to relax and center your focus.
- If you feel comfortable, proceed with the exercise.
- With your eyes closed, visualize the room you are in, including the walls, ceiling, and floor.
- Concentrate on recalling as many details as possible, from the arrangement of furniture to the colors of the walls.
- Open your eyes and observe your surroundings, taking note of what you remembered and what you forgot.
- Repeat the exercise, aiming to recall more details with each repetition.

Benefits:

- Increases mindfulness and presence by tuning into sensory perceptions.
- Enhances cognitive function by stimulating memory recall and attention to detail.
- Promotes relaxation and stress relief through deep breathing and visualization techniques.
- Improves spatial awareness and perception of the environment, leading to greater engagement with surroundings.

WEEK 1

DAY 1

EXERCISE	DURATIONS/REPS
Visual Warm-Up	5 minutes
Sit to Stand	3 reps
Basic Toe Balance	6 reps
Tiptoe Balance	6 reps
Tiptoe Walk	7 steps forward and 5 steps backward
Toe to Knee Chair-Assisted	3 reps per leg

DAY 2

EXERCISE	DURATIONS/REPS
Improving Awareness Exercise	5 minutes
Toe-Heel balance	6 reps
Heel Walk	7 steps forward and 5 steps backward
Ankle Point and Flex	10 reps per leg
Single-Leg Balance	4 reps
Knee Flex and Lift	6 reps per leg

DAY 3

EXERCISE	DURATIONS/REPS
Improving Awareness Exercise	5 minutes
Sit to Stand	4 reps
Dynamic Lunge	3 reps per leg
Basic Leg Hold Balance Chair-assisted	3 reps
Back Leg Extensions	4 reps per leg
Side Leg Raise	6 reps per leg

DAY 4

EXERCISE	DURATIONS/REPS
Improving Awareness Exercise	5 minutes
Leg Lift	10 reps per leg
Baby Steps Walk	7 steps forward and 5 steps backward
March Steps	10 steps forward
Tiptoe Balance	6 reps
Advanced Leg Hold Balance Chair-assisted	3 reps

DAY 5

EXERCISE	DURATIONS/REPS
Improving Awareness Exercise	5 minutes
Sit to Stand	5 reps
Heel Walk	7 steps forward and 5 steps backward
Ankle Point and Flex	10 reps per leg
Single-Leg Balance	4 reps
Knee Flex and Lift	6 reps per leg

DAY 6

EXERCISE	DURATIONS/REPS
Improving Awareness Exercise	5 minutes
Basic Toe Balance	15 seconds per leg
Tiptoe Balance	6 reps
Tiptoe Walk	7 steps forward and 5 steps backward
Toe to Knee Chair-Assisted	3 reps per leg
Dynamic Lunge	3 reps per leg

DAY 7

EXERCISE	DURATIONS/REPS
Improving Awareness Exercise	5 minutes
Tiptoe Balance	6 reps
Heel Walking	15 steps forward and 15 steps backward
March Steps	10 steps forward
Leg Lift	6 reps per leg
Advanced Leg Hold Balance Chair-assisted	4 reps

WEEK 2

DAY 8	
EXERCISE	DURATIONS/REPS
Visual Warm-Up	5 minutes
Sit to Stand	3 reps
Baby Steps Walk	7 steps forward and 5 steps backward
Basic Leg Hold Balance	3 reps
Knee Flex and Lift	6 reps per leg
Dynamic Lunge	3 reps per leg

DAY 9	
EXERCISE	DURATIONS/REPS
Improving Awareness	5 minutes
Advanced Tiptoe Balance	6 reps
Advanced Toe Balance	6 reps
March Steps	10 steps forward
Toe to Knee Chair-Assisted	3 reps per leg
Ankle Point and Flex	10 reps per leg

DAY 10

EXERCISE	DURATIONS/REPS
Improving Awareness	5 minutes
Sit to Stand	3 reps
Advanced Leg Hold Balance	3 reps
Tiptoe Walk	7 steps forward and 5 steps backward
Advanced Leg Lift	10 reps per leg
Side Leg Raise	6 reps per leg

DAY 11

EXERCISE	DURATIONS/REPS
Improving Awareness	5 minutes
Basic Toe Balance	15 seconds per leg
Tiptoe Balance	6 reps
Advanced Single-Leg Balance	4 reps
Toe to Knee Chair-Assisted	3 reps per leg
Dynamic Lunge	3 reps per leg

DAY 12

EXERCISE	DURATIONS/REPS
Improving Awareness	5 minutes
Toe-Heel balance	7 reps
Heel Walk	7 steps forward and 5 steps backward
Ankle Point and Flex	10 reps per leg
Advanced Single-Leg Balance	4 reps
Knee Flex and Lift	7 reps per leg

DAY 13

EXERCISE	DURATIONS/REPS
Improving Awareness	5 minutes
Advanced Tiptoe Balance	6 reps
Side Leg Raise:	6 reps per leg
March Steps	10 reps forward
Toe to Knee Chair-Assisted	6 reps per leg
Ankle Point and Flex	14 reps per leg

DAY 14

EXERCISE	DURATIONS/REPS
Improving Awareness	5 minutes
Sit to Stand	3 reps
Advanced Leg Hold Balance	5 reps
Tiptoe Walk	8 steps forward and 6 steps backward
Advanced Leg Lift	10 reps per leg
Side Leg Raise	6 reps per leg

WEEK 3

DAY 15

EXERCISE	DURATIONS/REPS
Improving Awareness	5 minutes
Sit to Stand	3 reps
Basic Toe Balance	6 reps
Advanced Tiptoe Balance	6 reps
Tiptoe Walk	8 steps forward and 6 steps backward
Toe to Knee	4 reps per leg

DAY 16

EXERCISE	DURATIONS/REPS
Visual Warm-Up	5 minutes
Toe-Heel balance	6 reps
Heel Walk	7 steps forward and 5 steps backward
Ankle Point and Flex	10 reps per leg
Advanced Single-Leg Balance	4 reps
Knee Flex and Lift	6 reps per leg

DAY 17

EXERCISE	DURATIONS/REPS
Improving Awareness Exercise	5 minutes
Sit to Stand	4 reps
Dynamic Lunge	4 reps per leg
Basic Leg Hold Balance	6 reps
Back Leg Extensions	4 reps per leg
Side Leg Raise	8 reps per leg

DAY 18

EXERCISE	DURATIONS/REPS
Visual Warm-Up	5 minutes
Baby Steps Walk	9 steps forward and 7 steps backward
Advanced Leg Lift	10 reps per leg
March Steps	10 steps forward
Advanced Tiptoe Balance	6 reps
Advanced Leg Hold Balance	9 reps

DAY 19

EXERCISE	DURATIONS/REPS
Improving Awareness Exercise	5 minutes
Sit to Stand	5 reps
Heel Walk	10 steps forward and 8 steps backward
Ankle Point and Flex	10 reps per leg
Advanced Single-Leg Balance	5 reps
Knee Flex and Lift	6 reps per leg

DAY 20

EXERCISE	DURATIONS/REPS
Improving Awareness Exercise	5 minutes
Advanced Toe Balance	6 reps
Advanced Tiptoe Balance	8 reps
Tiptoe Walk	10 steps forward and 8 steps backward
Toe to Knee	3 reps per leg
Dynamic Lunge	4 reps per leg

DAY 21

EXERCISE	DURATIONS/REPS
Visual Warm-Up	5 minutes
Advanced Tiptoe Balance	8 reps
Heel Walking	10 steps forward and 8 steps backward
March Steps	12 steps forward
Advanced Leg Lift	10 reps per leg
Advanced Leg Hold Balance	7 reps

WEEK 4

DAY 22	
EXERCISE	DURATIONS/REPS
Improving Awareness Exercise	5 minutes
Sit to Stand	3 reps
Basic Toe Balance	6 reps
Advanced Tiptoe Balance	6 reps
Tiptoe Walk	7 steps forward and 5 steps backward
Toe to Knee	6 reps per leg

DAY 23	
EXERCISE	DURATIONS/REPS
Visual Warm-Up	5 minutes
Toe-Heel balance	8 reps
Heel Walk	10 reps per leg
Ankle Point and Flex	10 reps per leg
Advanced Single-Leg Balance	8 reps
Knee Flex and Lift	8 reps per leg

DAY 24

EXERCISE	DURATIONS/REPS
Improving Awareness Exercise	5 minutes
Sit to Stand	4 reps
Dynamic Lunge	5 reps per leg
Basic Leg Hold Balance	4 reps
Back Leg Extensions	5 reps per leg
Side Leg Raise	8 reps per leg

DAY 25

EXERCISE	DURATIONS/REPS
Visual Warm-Up	5 minutes
Baby Steps Walk	12 steps forward and 10 steps backward
Advanced Leg Lift	12 reps per leg
March Steps	12 steps forward
Advanced Tiptoe Balance	4 reps
Advanced Leg Hold Balance	4 reps

DAY 26

EXERCISE	DURATIONS/REPS
Improving Awareness Exercise	5 minutes
Sit to Stand	5 reps
Heel Walk	12 steps forward and 8 steps backward
Ankle Point and Flex	12 reps per leg
Advanced Single-Leg Balance	10 reps
Knee Flex and Lift	10 reps per leg

DAY 27

EXERCISE	DURATIONS/REPS
Improving Awareness Exercise	5 minutes
Advanced Toe Balance	6 reps
Advanced Tiptoe Balance	6 reps
Tiptoe Walk	7 steps forward and 5 steps backward
Toe to Knee	3 reps per leg
Dynamic Lunge	3 reps per leg

DAY 28

EXERCISE	DURATIONS/REPS
Visual Warm-Up	5 minutes
Advanced Tiptoe Balance	6 reps
Heel Walking	10 reps per leg
March Steps	10 reps per leg
Advanced Leg Lift	10 reps per leg
Advanced Leg Hold Balance	4 reps

Following the completion of the 28-day balance exercise plan, it's important to hear from participants about their journey and experiences. Here are some insightful testimonials from individuals who have embarked on this program:

• Emily, 73: "Before starting the balance exercise plan, I often felt unsteady on my feet and lacked confidence in my movements. However, as I progressed through the program, I noticed a remarkable improvement in my balance and stability. Now, I feel much more secure in my ability to navigate daily activities without fear of falling."

• David, 81: "Initially, I was skeptical about the effectiveness of balance exercises, but I decided to give it a try due to persistent issues with mobility. To my surprise, I've experienced significant progress in my coordination and strength, particularly in my legs and core. Now, I feel more empowered and capable of moving with ease and grace."

• Emma, 79: "One of my biggest concerns before starting the balance exercise plan was my fear of falling, especially when playing with my grandchildren. However, after dedicating myself to the exercises, I've noticed a newfound sense of confidence and security in my movements. I no longer worry about losing my balance and can enjoy precious moments with my family without hesitation."

These testimonials highlight the positive impact of balance exercises on individuals' confidence, mobility, and overall well-being. Through dedication and perseverance, participants have overcome challenges and embraced a more active and fulfilling lifestyle.

Conclusion

As we conclude our journey through the balance exercises for seniors, let's take a moment to reflect on the profound impact these practices have had on our well-being. This book has served as a comprehensive guide, offering a holistic approach to integrating our mental, emotional, and physical selves.

Throughout the chapters, we've delved into exercises aimed at improving balance, enhancing stability, and fostering a deeper connection with our bodies. Each exercise builds upon the other, contributing to a sense of harmony and equilibrium within ourselves.

A central theme of this book has been the recognition of the mind-body connection. By engaging in these exercises, we've learned to deepen our awareness of our bodies and respond to them with compassion. This heightened awareness not only enhances our physical health but also profoundly impacts our mental and emotional well-being.

Moreover, the journey through these exercises has taught us valuable lessons in patience, mindfulness, and self-acceptance. We've discovered that consistent practice is key to achieving lasting results, and integrating other aspects of well-being, such as nutrition and hydration, enhances the effectiveness of our efforts.

These balance exercises are not just temporary fixes but lifelong companions, adaptable to all stages of life. They offer a pathway to emotional balance, physical relief, and heightened self-awareness. By engaging in them, we empower ourselves to take an active role in our own well-being.

In essence, the balance exercises for seniors provide opportunities for personal growth and restoration. May your journey lead you to serenity, equilibrium, and profound inner connection. We hope the insights gained from this book support you in leading a more wholesome, peaceful, and balanced life.

Aging is a natural aspect of life that shouldn't cause undue worry.
Let's embrace the beauty of each stage of life and courageously confront the obstacles that come our way. It's time to step forward with renewed confidence and face the future head-on.

Thank you for choosing my book.

I really would like to hear your thoughts about your experience because your input is valuable and can inspire those who want to start this rewarding journey.
If you have a moment, please consider leaving a review.

Printed in Great Britain
by Amazon